STO

37

3.15.78

THE EPILEPSY
FACT BOOK

THE EPILEPSY FACT BOOK

Harry Sands, PhD

Director of Research
Postgraduate Center for Mental Health
New York, New York
and
Consultant
Epilepsy Foundation of America
Washington, D. C.

Frances C. Minters

Consultant
Epilepsy Foundation of America
Washington, D. C.

SPONSORED BY EPILEPSY FOUNDATION OF AMERICA

 F. A. DAVIS COMPANY / PHILADELPHIA

Printed in the United States of America

Library of Congress Cataloging in Publication Data

Sands, Harry.
   The epilepsy fact book.

   Bibliography: p.
   Includes index.
   1. Epilepsy. I. Minters, Frances C., joint author. II. Title.
[DNLM: 1. Epilepsy—Popular works. WL385 S221]
RC372.S257   616.8′53   77-24279
ISBN 0-8036-7725-1

This book is dedicated to Paul E. Funk, former Executive Vice-President and Past President of the Epilepsy Foundation of America.

Foreword

This is a book that I have long wanted to see written. It is, essentially, a book for lay readers, written in lay terms. The book addresses itself not to those subjects which are important to physicians and other professionals, but rather to those subjects that are important to the person who has epilepsy, and that person's family, friends, employers—all those whose lives are touched by this most misunderstood of physical disorders.

There are numerous medical texts written by doctors, psychiatrists, psychologists, and other professionals in the field. This book does not seek to duplicate those excellent references. Rather, it strives to fill an entirely different need.

Books addressed to the professional, quite understandably, tend to emphasize epilepsy as a disease or disorder, concentrating on what it is, how it came to be, how it physically affects the individual, how it can be medically controlled. This book emphasizes epilepsy as an illness—meaning, how do you live with it? How do you cope with the social and psychologic conditions that affect the person with epilepsy and all those around that person? In essence, how does that person learn to live a full, normal, productive life? And how do those around him contribute to that growth?

The authors have done a superb job of presenting a complex and multifaceted subject. However, persons with epilepsy and the parents of children with epilepsy have also shared in the writing of this book. For the subjects discussed here are those which have been raised over and over again by the hundreds of thousands of persons, of all races, all ages, and all socioeconomic levels, who have written to the Epilepsy Foundation of America headquarters over the past few years.

The questions answered here are those which may be thought of after the person has left the doctor's office or those which people may hesitate to ask the doctor—questions which deserve detailed, empathetic answers.

The material reflects the deep understanding of epilepsy possessed by the authors. Harry Sands has been devoted to the cause of persons with epilepsy for more than a quarter of a century.

It is my sincere hope that this book finds its way into all of the two million homes where the life of a family has been touched by this disorder. People with epilepsy can and must be their own best friend, their own best advocate. And this book should help many attain that goal.

Paul E. Funk
Former Executive Vice-President and
Past President
Epilepsy Foundation of America

Preface

Despite the success of ongoing medical and scientific research in controlling seizures, the experiences of epilepsy can still immerce persons with epilepsy, their families, and their communities in a whirlpool of negative feelings. This book is written in the hope of dispelling the confusions and subduing the unrealistic fears and anxieties.

We are grateful to the Epilepsy Foundation of America, whose support and encouragement made this book a reality. The Foundation's staff was continuously helpful, and Dr. Leonard G. Perlman, Lewis A. Strudler, and Executive Director Jack McAllister, who guided the project to completion, deserve our special thanks. The Foundation's professional advisory board, and especially Dr. Cesare T. Lombroso, chairman of its publications committee, gave us much helpful advice.

We also thank Dr. Richard L. Masland, who served as our medical advisor, and whose vast knowledge and deep concern for persons with epilepsy was ever there to guide us.

Our special thanks go to Paul E. Funk, former Executive Vice-President and Past President of the Foundation, for his support, enthusiasm, and his numerous creative suggestions.

HS
FCM

Contents

1

The Nature of Epilepsy

WHAT IS EPILEPSY?

Suddenly you are confronted with an unexpected situation. You or someone close to you has epilepsy. The condition used to seem strange and remote, but now it has happened to you. You want to find out all you can about epilepsy. Fifty years ago, this in itself would have been a problem. You could have collected a lot of rumors and unfounded ideas about epilepsy, but few real facts. Today we are more fortunate.

Modern medical thinking about epilepsy started in the mid-nineteenth century. An English doctor, John Hughlings Jackson, was one of its pioneers.

Long before Jackson's time—around 400 B.C., in fact—the Greek physician Hippocrates correctly identified the brain as the organ involved in epilepsy. Many of Hippocrates' contemporaries, however, continued to attribute epilepsy to supernatural causes. These beliefs continued through the Middle Ages, when most people believed that epilepsy was caused by demons. Although many physicians of the time stayed with Hippocrates' view, their anatomic knowledge was sketchy, their ideas of how the brain worked were largely mistaken, and they could not substantiate their opinions of what caused epilepsy.

In the nineteenth century, the study of brain function advanced rapidly. As far as epilepsy was concerned, the high point of research was reached in 1870, when Jackson identified the cerebral cortex, the brain's outer layer, as the part involved in epilepsy. Jackson also described how nerve cells trigger epileptic seizures.

Since Jackson's time, many scientists have carried on the work of identifying the functions of the various parts of the brain. Although the work has not yet been completed, we know more about how the brain works than even our parents did. This research has helped us understand epilepsy.

Anatomy of the Brain

The human brain is a marvelously complicated organ; it has to be, for it controls every waking and sleeping activity, every conscious and unconscious thought and need and process that we engage in.

A part of the human brain that is essential for our thinking and intelligence is the cerebral cortex, the upper surface of the brain. The cerebral cortex is comprised of soft tissue known as the "gray matter." The gray matter is intricately folded in order to increase the surface area of the brain. It resembles a crumpled sheet of paper. If it were smoothed out, it would be about three feet long and two feet wide. The cerebral cortex covers the cerebrum, the major portion of the brain.

The cerebrum is divided into areas called "lobes." The lobes are separated by large depressions, or fissures. Each lobe is responsible for various functions—for example, the occipital lobe, at the back of the brain, is concerned with vision.

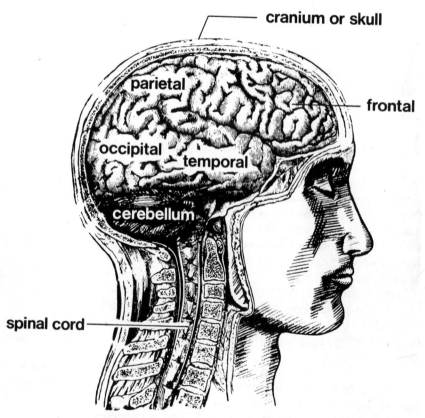

The brain (modified from picture furnished by The Bettmann Archive).

Beneath the cerebrum is a specialized part of the brain called the cerebellum. The cerebellum monitors and modulates body movements. Below the cerebellum is the brain stem, which connects with the spinal cord. Through the spinal cord, nerve fibers transmit impulses between the brain and other regions of the body.

The brain and the spinal cord together are called the central nervous system (often referred to as the CNS).

Nerve Cells

The nerve cells, or neurons, are part of the tissue forming the central nervous system. Altogether, there are about 10 billion neurons in the brain and spinal cord.

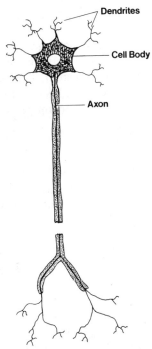

A neuron (Mark Schnapper, Abramson Studio).

Each neuron has three parts: the cell body, the dendrites, and the axon. Dendrites are fibers with many branches. They serve as receivers. Their function is to pick up electrical impulses that are transmitted from other cells. Axons, which form the long "tail" of the nerve, serve as the transmitters. Their function is to pass on information, in the form of electrical impulses, to other cells. The electrochemical reactions by which the brain operates take place within the cell body itself.

3

How Does the Brain Work?

The central nervous system is an electrochemical system. The sense organs—eyes, ears, nose, tastebuds, skin (for touch)—receive information about the environment, but they do not interpret it. They pass the raw data along to the brain. The information travels in the form of electrical impulses. The brain interprets these impulses. Based on its interpretation, it then relays instructions for action to the body. These instructions are also in the form of electrical impulses. The responsibility for transmitting these electronic messages back and forth rests with the nerve cells, the neurons.

Neurons live in a fluid that is electrically charged with chemical particles called ions. Inside the cell body there are ions, too; they have a different electrical charge. When a neuron is appropriately stimulated, its cell wall suddenly becomes porous. The ion particles outside flow in. The meeting of the two types of ions sets off an electrical charge, and the neuron discharges, or fires an electrical inpulse.

When one neuron fires, the electrical charge thus set up may spread to a neighboring neuron. It fires, too. In this way, impulses travel from one neuron to another along the nervous system. This complicated process all takes place in a thousandth of a second or less, although the transmission of the nerve impulses may be as slow as 0.1 meter per second.

Sometimes Something Goes Wrong

Neurons are information processors as well as transmitters and receivers. The world is full of stimuli, and if all the insignificant information our senses received were passed on indiscriminately, our brains would be, quite simply, flooded; we would be incapable of action.

One of the functions of neurons is to block useless information. This inhibition, too, works electrochemically. When the voltage difference between the ions entering the cell and those already there is high, the impulse is inhibited and the neuron does not fire. Or rather, this is what should happen. Sometimes it does not.

Occasionally, the inhibitory function of a few neurons is disrupted. Under certain circumstances, the neurons appear to lose their ability to function in an independent fashion. Groups of neurons develop an abnormal rhythmic synchronous discharge. Like soldiers walking in step across a bridge, large forces develop. In the brain, this takes the form of high-voltage electrical discharges of groups of neurons. These discharges are self-perpetuating, and their spread along the pathways of the brain is an essential feature of the epileptic seizure. As Jackson put it, "Epilepsy is the name for occasional, sudden, excessive, rapid and local discharges of grey matter."*

---

*Jackson, J. H.: *Selected Writings, vol. I.* Basic Books, New York, 1958.

4

It does not take much to cause an epileptic disturbance. There are 10 billion neurons in the central nervous system. If as few as seven of them malfunction at the same time, a seizure may result.

The Brain Is Like an Orchestra

When the brain is functioning properly, it acts asynchronously, that is, at many levels at once. It can receive messages through all the senses and transmit instructions to many parts of the body at the same time. A person can simultaneously see, hear, smell, walk, and talk. This is because each part of the brain works separately, and at the same time all the parts act together to produce an integrated human being.

When the brain is doing its job in this way, it is like a well-conducted orchestra. In an orchestra each section—brass, strings, woodwinds—plays independently, yet all combine to produce a harmonious pattern of sound. But suppose something suddenly goes wrong in the brass section, and the brasses can now sound only one note—one loud note. The rest of the orchestra momentarily loses track of the score. For the moment, the whole orchestra sounds the same one note. The orchestra has become synchronous.

Something like that happens to the brain in an epileptic seizure. Suddenly a small section of neurons takes over, and the whole brain becomes temporarily synchronous; it can sound only one note. For the moment, no other messages can get through. And the person experiences a seizure.

Brain Waves

In 1929 a German physician, Hans Berger, demonstrated that the electrical impulses that are transmitted by the human brain can be measured from outside the skull and recorded. This knowledge was used to develop the electroencephalograph (EEG), a machine that shows the shape, voltage, and frequency of the electrical impulses, which are called brain waves.

The electroencephalograph has made it possible to see the excessive

normal

wave and spike 3 sec.

1 sec.

Electroencephalograms of normal and spike-and-wave brain wave patterns (modified from recordings furnished by Dr. Eli Goldensohn).

discharge of the neurons in the brain that typically takes place in epilepsy. In petit mal seizures, for example, the EEG shows that the neurons are discharging in a pattern called the three-per-second spike-and-wave. A nonseizure brain wave pattern and a spike-and-wave pattern are shown in the picture on page 5.

Is There Always a Brain Injury in Epilepsy?

In some cases of epilepsy, physicians can demonstrate that a part of the brain has been injured and that this injured section is probably responsible for the seizures. In many other cases of epilepsy, physicians cannot pinpoint an injury. For some persons, epilepsy may merely represent some constitutional or "built in" overreactivity of the brain.

Other Brain Disorders

There are, of course, many other brain disorders besides epilepsy. Whether an injury in the brain will cause epilepsy or some other disorder depends on which part of the brain is affected and on the nature of the trouble spot.

What Next?

Researchers are still working on methods of pinpointing the brain and nerve mechanisms responsible for the symptoms of epilepsy, especially the processes that cause the uncontrolled overactivity of neurons in seizures. Once the causes are identified precisely, we'll be that much closer to an improved diagnosis and a definite cure.

WHAT HAPPENS DURING A SEIZURE?

What do you think of when you hear the word "seizure"? To most people, the word conjures up images of a person falling unconscious to the ground. Some seizures are like that, but not all. Some seizures are very undramatic. Some, in fact, go entirely unnoticed, even by the person involved. Depending on the type of epilepsy, the only sign of a seizure may be a fleeting interruption of consciousness, a twitching limb, an aching stomach, or even, occasionally, a headache.

Seizures, however, are not necessarily equivalent to epilepsy. Seizures may also be caused by something *external* to the brain itself. For example, seizures may result from low blood sugar (hypoglycemia) or from a number of other toxic, metabolic disorders.

The word "epilepsy" comes from the Greek word for seizure, and seizures are the major symptoms of epilepsy. They are symptoms of the brain's temporary burst of abnormal activity, expressed through altered control over some part of the body. The kind of seizure that occurs depends upon which part of the brain is the seat of the abnormal electrical discharge, how many brain cells are involved, and how long the discharge lasts.

Types of Seizures

Epilepsy is usually classified by the type of seizure the person has. Seizures used to be described as grand mal, petit mal, psychomotor, and so on. Most physicians now prefer to use the International Classification System, which describes seizures in relation to the area of the brain involved.

The new system divides seizures into two main groups: partial and generalized. The difference is that generalized seizures involve the entire brain; partial seizures affect only part of the brain. There are also unilateral seizures, which affect only one side, or hemisphere, of the brain.

Although we'll continue to use the older, more familiar names for seizures in our discussion, for your reference the newer names are provided below.

International Classification of Seizure Types*

I. Partial Seizures (seizures which involve or begin in one area of the brain).
   A. Partial seizures with elementary symptomatology (seizures that have relatively uncomplicated symptoms. Usually the person remains conscious).
      1. With motor symptoms (symptoms affecting the muscles).
      2. With sensory or somatosensory symptoms (symptoms affecting the senses).
      3. With autonomic symptoms (symptoms affecting the internal organs).
      4. Compound forms (symptoms of more than one of the above types).
   B. Partial seizures with complex symptomatology (partial seizures with more complicated symptoms, usually with some loss of consciousness).
      1. With impairment of consciousness only.
      2. With cognitive symptomatology (symptoms affecting thought).
      3. With affective symptomatology (symptoms affecting mood or emotion).
      4. With "psychosensory" symptomatology (symptoms affecting sense perception, such as illusions or hallucinations).

---

*Gastaut, H.: *Clinical and electroencephalographical classification of epileptic seizures.* Epilepsia 11:102, 1970. Material in parentheses added.

5. With "psychomotor" symptomatology (symptoms such as movement and behavior inappropriate to the situation).
6. Compound forms (symptoms of more than one of the above types).

C. Partial seizures secondarily generalized (seizures that begin as partial seizures and then become generalized).

II. Generalized Seizures (seizures that involve both sides of the brain).
   A. Absences (brief lapses of consciousness occurring without warning and unaccompanied by prominent movements, as in petit mal).
   B. Bilateral massive epileptic myoclonus (an involuntary jerking contraction of the major muscles).
   C. Infantile spasms (brief muscle spasms in young children).
   D. Clonic seizures (seizures consisting of jerking movements of the muscles).
   E. Tonic seizures (seizures in which the muscles are rigid).
   F. Tonic-clonic seizures (seizures which begin with muscle rigidity and progress to jerking muscular movement, commonly known as "grand mal" seizures).
   G. Atonic seizures (seizures in which there is a loss of muscle tone and the person falls to the ground).
   H. Akinetic seizures (seizures in which there is a loss of muscle movement).

III. Unilateral Seizures (seizures involving one hemisphere, or half, of the brain and consequently affecting one side of the body).

IV. Unclassified Epileptic Seizures (seizures which, because of incomplete information, cannot be put in a category).

Petit Mal

Petit mal (one of the group of generalized seizures, according to the International Classification System) usually has its onset during childhood. The seizures consist of periods of altered consciousness. The child temporarily "blacks out" during a seizure. The blackout is short—typically, it lasts from 5 to 30 seconds—and has its onset without warning.

When you see a person having a petit mal seizure, you might think he is just staring blankly into space for a few seconds. Sometimes the child's eyes seem to roll back into his head. There may be slight, rhythmic movements of the facial muscles, the head, or the arms. When the seizure is over, the child usually goes on with whatever he was doing before it began. He does not know that he blacked out; he has no recall of what happened during the seizure.

There is no set rule about how often petit mal seizures occur. A person may have as many as fifty or even a hundred a day—or as few as one or two a month.

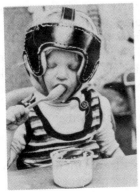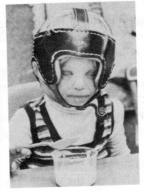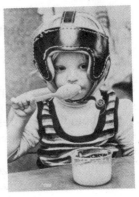

Child during petit mal seizure. Note protective helmet.

Grand Mal

Grand mal is what most people think epilepsy is all about. In terms of the International Classification, these seizures are a part of the generalized group; like petit mal, they involve the entire brain.

A grand mal seizure begins with a sudden loss of consciousness. The person falls stiffly to the ground, sometimes uttering a birdlike cry as he does so. Because his breathing is temporarily interrupted, his skin may turn a pale, bluish color. Then his whole body starts to jerk. Breathing resumes but is heavy and irregular. During this phase, the individual may bite his tongue, and he may involuntarily lose bladder control. Soon the shaking movements stop, and the person relaxes. To an onlooker, a seizure may seem endless; but it seldom lasts longer than two or three minutes.

After the seizure, some people are able to resume their normal activities within a few minutes; others feel drowsy, confused, weak, nauseated, restless, or irritable for some time. Headaches are common. Some people require a short nap. Although people are generally unconscious during a grand mal seizure, they are usually aware, afterwards, that they have had one; this is because their muscles are sore from all the shaking.

Psychomotor Seizures

Psychomotor seizures (called partial seizures with complex symptoms, in the International Classification System) are often caused by a disturbance in the temporal lobe of the brain (see the illustration of the brain on page 2).

At the beginning of a psychomotor seizure, a person may become dizzy for no apparent reason, or confused, or afraid, or angry. He may experience strange sensations—a ringing in his ears, spots before his eyes, changes in the way he sees colors. At first, the person is usually not completely unconscious; but his state of awareness is affected to some extent. His sense of time may be distorted; he may not know where he is; his sense of self-identity may become clouded. His own home may seem suddenly unfamiliar to him, or he may feel at home in a stranger's place.

Later, there is a state of impaired awareness during which some people perform purposeless motions known as "automatisms." They may walk aimlessly, smack their lips, stare blankly into space, grimace, rub their hands or legs, or pick at or unbutton their clothes.

Psychomotor seizures may last only for a minute, or they may go on for several hours. Frequently, a psychomotor seizure progresses into a generalized convulsion.

Usually, after the seizure is over, the person falls asleep. Often he cannot remember what happened; it is as if the whole episode took place in a dream.

Jacksonian Seizures

Jacksonian seizures (a type of partial seizure) are named after John Hughlings Jackson, who first described them in the 1870s.

This type of seizure occurs most often in adults. The attack begins with an involuntary jerking movement in some part of the body, usually an extremity—for example, the thumb and forefinger, the toes—or the mouth or tongue. The individual is usually conscious during this part of the seizure, which generally lasts only a short while—a few seconds or minutes. But then, sometimes, the spasms spread throughout the whole body (this phenomenon is called the "Jacksonian march") and a grand mal seizure, with loss of consciousness, follows.

Autonomic Seizures

Autonomic seizures (another type of partial seizure) affect the autonomic nervous system which controls involuntary body functions such as digestion and heartbeat. These seizures do not involve the whole brain, nor do they produce unconsciousness. Their symptoms are headaches that happen again and again without apparent cause, stomachaches, nausea, vomiting, or fever. Of course, these symptoms also occur in a great many other conditions. Only a thorough physical examination can show whether they are caused by epilepsy.

Unilateral Seizures

Sometimes during infancy there occurs an unusual type of attack in which only one side of the body is affected. The facial muscles, arm muscles, or leg muscles on one side twitch violently, while those on the other side remain under control. This type of seizure is called a unilateral seizure. Sometimes in a unilateral seizure the muscles on both sides of the body are affected, but more so on one side than on the other. The individual is usually conscious during a unilateral seizure.

Infantile Spasms

Repeated attacks of convulsive movements in babies and very young children are called infantile spasms. In this type of seizure, the arms, the body, and sometimes the head suddenly jerk violently forward. These jerks are extremely brief, but they may recur several times a day.

Other Kinds of Seizures

There are still other kinds of seizures. There are clonic seizures, in which the body jerks rapidly. There are tonic seizures, in which the body is unnaturally rigid (grand mal seizures have both a tonic and a clonic phase). And there is bilateral massive epileptic myoclonus, which consists of involuntary muscle movements involving the whole body—"myoclonus," in fact, means muscle jerks. But all these seizures are rarer than the ones that we have described in detail.

Percentage of People with Different Types of Seizures

Most people have only one type of epilepsy. There are some, though, who have two or more types of seizures; and some people have one type of seizure at one period of their lives and another type later on.

To find out what percentage of people have each type of epilepsy, French researchers recently made a study of 6,000 private epilepsy patients. Almost a quarter of these cases could not be classified. The remainder were classified as shown in the table below.

Occurrence of Different Types of Seizures

Classification	Percentage of classified cases
Generalized epilepsy	37.7
Primary generalized epilepsy	28.4
Grand mal	11.3
Petit Mal	9.9
Myoclonus	4.1
Other	3.2
Secondary generalized epilepsy	9.3
Partial epilepsy	62.3
Elementary symptomatology	10.0
Complex symptomatology (psychomotor)	39.7
Secondarily generalized seizures	12.6

(Data from Gastaut, H., et al.: *Relative frequency of different types of epilepsy: A study employing the classification of the International League Against Epilepsy.* Epilepsia 16:459, Sept., 1975.)

What Is a Febrile Convulsion?

Not every seizure is caused by epilepsy. Other things can cause seizures, too; and in children under the age of five, a common cause of seizures is fever.

When they are running a high temperature, young children often go into convulsions. They are a common disorder of childhood. In fact, "febrile seizures are perhaps the most common neurologic disorder in childhood," reports Dr. Sidney Carter, Professor of Neurology at the College of Physicians and Surgeons of Columbia University, and chief of the division of pediatric neurology at Columbia-Presbyterian Medical Center.

If your child has a convulsion, call your doctor. He will take steps to prevent it from happening again.

What Is an Aura?

Sometimes the more recognizable symptoms of a seizure are preceded by a set of symptoms called the "aura."

There are many types of auras. Usually, they come in the form of sensations. A person may notice a ringing sound in his ears, a strange smell in his nostrils, or a crawling feeling on his skin. He may become giddy, or queasy in the stomach. He may suddenly become frightened without any apparent reason, or just have a vague feeling that something is wrong.

Although there are many different types of auras, usually an individual with epilepsy has the same aura every time he is about to have a seizure. Many people have learned to recognize these warning signs that a seizure is beginning. Some of them try to ward off the attack; others have enough time between the aura and the rest of the seizure to move to a quiet or safe place.

However, the aura is not a reliable warning for everybody. Only about 50 percent of people with epilepsy have an aura at all—and even these people do not have one every time. Besides, for many people the aura is not a warning, but actually part of the seizure itself; the aura symptoms are so quickly followed by unconsciousness that the person has no time to do anything at all about it.

Seizure Triggers

Why does a person with epilepsy have a seizure at one particular time and not at another? Basically, it depends on the state of the brain cells; but sometimes we can also identify something outside the person that sets off the seizure.

These outside triggers vary from person to person. Almost anything can be a seizure trigger for somebody. For example, some seizures are set off by a sound of a certain pitch, and others by a light that flickers at a particular frequency.

If a person with epilepsy and his doctor establish what his seizure triggers are, then the person can avoid these things. For most people, however, this solution is not possible, because for them there is no one factor that sets off a seizure each and every time.

Do People Lose Consciousness During a Seizure?

With the most common types of seizure, there is some loss of consciousness.

In a petit mal seizure, the person is usually unconscious for less than 30 seconds.

In a grand mal seizure, the person is usually unconscious for only one or two minutes; occasionally, the loss of consciousness may extend for as long as five minutes.

When a person is unconscious, he is not aware of what is taking place. He is not embarrassed. He cannot feel pain. To onlookers, the person undergoing a grand mal seizure may appear to be suffering. After all, his facial expression is distorted, and all his muscles are violently twitching. But these things are caused by the person's temporary loss of muscle control, not by feelings of distress. The person is not in pain. The movements do not hurt.

How to Help

It is only natural to want to help anybody in trouble, and a person who is having a grand mal attack certainly seems to be suffering. That's why it's important to remember that actually he is not in pain, nor, usually, in danger.

The main rule for helpers is to keep calm. Remember that there is nothing you or anyone else can do to stop a seizure once it has started.

Let the seizure run its course. Do not try to hold the person down or to restrain his movements in any way. It does help to loosen any tight clothing he may be wearing—to undo his belt and his tie, for example. You can also clear the area around him so that he cannot hurt himself by slamming into a hard object. Roll up your jacket or sweater or something else that's soft and place it under his head for a pillow. If you can do it gently and without too much strain, turn the person on his side so that excess saliva—which is caused by lack of muscle control—can flow freely from his mouth.

Do not try to open the person's mouth or to force anything between his teeth. If his mouth is already open, you might place a soft object, such as a folded handkerchief, between the side teeth to keep him from biting his tongue. Remember that this is not essential; a person cannot swallow his tongue. He may bite it—and this will make his saliva bloody—but the bite is hardly ever severe enough to do any great damage. There is much more

13

danger of injury if his helpers put hard objects in his mouth. As Helen Kitchen Branson, a nurse who herself has epilepsy, says:

> I have had pencils shoved through the roof of my mouth, pills poked down my throat until I nearly choked to death, water poured over me until I gasped for breath. In danger of dying from an epileptic seizure? Never. . . . In danger of dying from choking or drowning because well-meaning souls wanted to "help"? Many times.*

The rules given above are for grand mal seizures; but many of them also apply to giving aid during a psychomotor seizure. The first thing to remember is that you cannot shorten the seizure by your actions, and you should be careful not to grab the individual or try to restrain him. Someone in a psychomotor seizure may lash out in an unconscious, instinctive reaction to restraints. Shouting or telling him loudly to wake up can have the same result—and it will not speed the end of the seizure. Let him be.

After either a grand mal or a psychomotor seizure, someone should stay with the person until he has recovered consciousness completely and is no longer confused. Treat the incident in a calm, matter-of-fact way. People with epilepsy appreciate this. They are embarrassed when they see a lot of frightened people around them after a seizure.

Let the person rest until he feels well again, and then let him go on with his regular activities. He usually does not need any further care.

Is Medical Care Necessary in a Seizure?

It is usually not necessary to call a doctor or an ambulance when a person is having a seizure. Most often, he will recover from the attack without medical care.

There are two situations, though, that do call for medical attention—fast. Call a doctor or an ambulance at once if: (1) the seizure lasts for more than 10 minutes; or (2) there is a series of grand mal attacks, one following another in rapid succession. Either of these conditions is known as "status epilepticus."

Status epilepticus is an unusual condition but a dangerous one. Long, continued, or repeated seizures become increasingly difficult to stop, and if permitted to continue indefinitely, may lead to exhaustion and even death. The condition can be brought on if a person suddenly stops taking anticonvulsant medications. It is treated by intravenous injections of anticonvulsants.

Status epilepticus is a medical emergency. Anyone undergoing continuous grand mal seizures must be taken to a hospital at once.

---

*Branson, H. K.: *The epileptic: How you can help.* RN Magazine 35:48, 1972.

Are There Any Aftereffects?

The occurrence of aftereffects depends on the type of seizure. Minor seizures, such as those of petit mal or psychomotor attacks, appear to have little if any residual effects. Severe grand mal seizures, especially if they are prolonged, as in status epilepticus, may be associated with rather prolonged periods of asphyxia, a condition in which the body does not get enough oxygen. Frequently repeated seizures of this sort over long periods of time may lead to some intellectual impairment.

Associated Problems of Persons with Epilepsy

It should be emphasized that epileptic seizures may be a symptom of many different forms of brain injury or disease. Some of these conditions may lead to impairment of brain function, such as retardation or mental illness. These other symptoms are *not*, however, an essential feature of epilepsy.

WHAT CAUSES EPILEPSY?

We said that nowadays we know a lot about epilepsy. And we do; but there is still a lot that we don't know. For example, we know that in epilepsy some brain cells discharge when they aren't supposed to. But we do not yet know why this happens. This is the basic and central question that must be answered before we can truly say that we know what causes epilepsy. Researchers are studying both the normal and abnormal functioning of brain cells, and hopefully before too long they will be able to identify the underlying causes of epilepsy.

Some events that cause epilepsy can already be identified, although we do not know why they make the brain react abnormally. We know that epilepsy may follow some injury that occurs before or during birth. We know that it may result from congenital malformations dating from before birth. Nutritional deficiencies, fever, certain diseases, brain tumors and abscesses, and head wounds can also lead to epilepsy. Probably any of these factors, when they are followed by epilepsy, have caused some injury to the nerve cells in the brain, or to the way the nerve cells interact with one another. But just what the injury is cannot always be identified.

When we can point to the cause of the epilepsy, the disorder is called "symptomatic" epilepsy. When no cause can be found, the disorder is termed "essential" or "idiopathic" epilepsy.

Who Gets Epilepsy?

Anyone, at any time, may experience an injury or disease of the brain or central nervous system that may lead to epilepsy.

15

Epilepsy is not more common in one sex, or one race, or one geographic area. It is true, though, that some people do not know where or how to obtain proper medical care. A lack of medical care may result in a higher rate of epilepsy, especially in epilepsy associated with birth injuries. Prenatal clinics and well-baby clinics are excellent places to obtain quality medical care that will prevent injuries which might cause epilepsy.

Birth and Before

Before birth, a child may suffer brain damage that can result in epilepsy. Several factors can cause this. Radiation is one danger; that is why doctors avoid giving x-rays to pregnant women. Poisonous substances, including drugs, are another factor. Brain damage can also result if the mother catches an infectious disease, such as German measles, in the early stages of pregnancy.

There are other developmental and inherited causes of epilepsy. The Rh factor used to be one of them, although it is no longer a problem to anyone receiving adequate medical care.

The Rh factor is an ingredient of the red blood cells. Most people have it—they are Rh-positive. About 15 percent of people, however, are Rh-negative. If an Rh-positive man and Rh-negative woman have a baby, the child may be Rh-positive, and the mother's blood may develop antibodies against the child's blood. The first child won't be affected by the reaction, but a second child may be born with erythroblastosis fetalis, or severe anemia. In anemia, the blood can't carry oxygen efficiently, and if the shortage of oxygen is severe, the brain is affected. But this kind of anemia can be prevented. Today, Rh-negative women are routinely given an injection right after they give birth to prevent the antibodies from forming.

Epilepsy may also be caused at birth. In a premature or difficult labor, the infant may be deprived of oxygen. Brain damage is always a risk when there is a shortage of oxygen, and brain damage may lead to epilepsy.

Sometimes the effects of a birth or prebirth injury are apparent at once. Sometimes they do not show up until later in life. If epilepsy is caused by a prenatal or natal injury, chances are the disorder will appear (1) before the age of five or (2) at puberty.

Childhood and After

After infancy, the factors that cause epilepsy to develop are varied. Until the end of the elementary school years, most epilepsy is an aftereffect of head injuries or childhood diseases such as measles, encephalitis, whooping cough, and meningitis. These diseases that may produce epilepsy are infectious; but epilepsy itself is not contagious.

In adults, epilepsy can be caused by brain tumors, blood circulation problems that limit the oxygen supply of the brain, or by head injuries. It's estimated that many thousands of people develop epilepsy each year following head injuries sustained in automobile accidents.

Can You Outgrow Epilepsy?

Parents often wonder if their child will outgrow his epilepsy. It's a natural question to ask, but a difficult one to answer.

Sometimes children do outgrow epilepsy. Under a doctor's guidance and with careful supervision, between 47 and 92 percent of children stop having seizures by the time they reach adolescence.*

On the other hand, for some people seizures intensify with age, occur for the first time in adulthood, become more frequent, or change from one type to another as a person grows older.

Still other people have the same type of epilepsy throughout their lives.

The picture is complicated, and what will happen in any individual case is hard to predict. But one thing seems certain—the sooner the diagnosis and the better the control, the greater is the chance of outgrowing the condition.

Is Epilepsy Inherited?

Suppose two people are in a car accident. They each suffer the same type of head injury. But one develops epilepsy, and the other doesn't. Why?

What may make the difference is each person's "seizure threshold," the susceptibility of each person's brain to the development of seizures. Is the seizure threshold inherited? Does heredity make some people more likely than others to develop epilepsy? All we can answer at the present time is that there are constitutional differences which may play a part in the individual's susceptibility.

Just as we inherit the color of our eyes, our hair, and our height, so we all may inherit a particular seizure threshold. But heredity alone is rarely, if ever, solely responsible for epilepsy. Research so far indicates that in most cases the interaction between heredity and environment is responsible. This is especially true in symptomatic epilepsy, where the factor that led to the development of epilepsy can be identified.

Sometimes epilepsy is caused by brain injury during pregnancy or during birth. These injuries are not inherited. Thus, the role of heredity in any person with epilepsy probably depends on the nature of his particular case.

People with epilepsy often ask whether they should have children. As noted above, the risk depends on the nature of the person's epilepsy. To make certain that the risks are as low as possible, couples with a history of

---

*Holowach, J., Thurston, D. L., and O'Leary, J.: *Prognosis in childhood epilepsy.* New England Journal of Medicine 286:169, Jan. 27, 1972.

epilepsy or brain defects in their families may be advised to consult a physician who specializes in genetic counseling before they decide to have a child. A genetic counselor can tell you if the risks to your baby will be great or slight.

However, in view of the many different conditions and diseases that can cause epilepsy, it is clear that it can happen to anybody. As Paul E. Funk, former executive vice-president of the Epilepsy Foundation of America, said, "We are all potentially epileptic, and epilepsy can indeed touch the life of anyone at any time."

An Ounce of Prevention

We cannot totally prevent epilepsy—not at this stage in our knowledge; but we can lessen our chances of getting it.

Proper medical care in pregnancy and childbirth are important steps toward preventing epilepsy. The chances of brain injury before, during, and after birth decrease with early and continuing medical supervision.

Fortunately for us, medical science is improving all the time. Every time scientists succeed in preventing an infectious disease that can injure the central nervous system, it automatically eliminates another source of epilepsy.

Good nutrition also plays a part in epilepsy prevention, although as far as we know the role is a minor one. Vitamin B_6 deficiencies and magnesium deficiencies can both cause seizures—but these are relatively uncommon causes. To guard against epilepsy, we need not dose ourselves with vitamins as long as we eat a well-balanced diet.

Our best protection against epilepsy is to prevent serious head injuries of all types. Motorcyclists, football players, horseback riders, construction workers, and others who wear helmets because of the danger of head injuries are protecting themselves against epilepsy. So are motorists who observe lower speed limits and drive carefully. One of the best protective devices of all is a securely fastened seat belt.

FACTS AND FIGURES

How Many People Have Epilepsy?

The most recent scientific studies indicate that about 0.6 percent of the population has had recurrent seizures within any 5-year period. Over 6 percent of the population has at least one seizure during their lifetime. The Epilepsy Foundation of America estimates that about 2 million Americans, or 1 percent of the population, have some form of epilepsy.

How Many New Cases Occur Each Year?

Statisticians estimate that there about a hundred thousand new cases of epilepsy each year.

At What Age Do People Get Epilepsy?

Epilepsy is not limited to a particular age group. About 75 percent of the cases occur before the age of 20; the other 25 percent occur at later stages of life.

What Effect Does Epilepsy Have on Life Expectancy?

We know that, except in the case of status epilepticus, people do not usually die from an epileptic seizure. As for the long-term effects of epilepsy, some statistics suggest that life expectancy may be slightly lower for persons with epilepsy than for persons without it; but with good medical care, the difference can be insignificant.

2

The Treatment of Epilepsy

HOW DO THEY KNOW IT'S EPILEPSY?

The sailors in *H.M.S. Pinafore* inform us that:

Things are seldom what they seem,
Skim milk masquerades as cream.*

And that's the way it is with epilepsy. Sometimes symptoms that seem like those of epilepsy turn out to be caused by something else; sometimes symptoms that seem atypical turn out to be a sign of epilepsy. The doctor's job is to get a complete picture of the patient's condition before he starts treatment.

What Brings the Patient to the Doctor?

There are some cases where a person sees a doctor when the symptoms of epilepsy first appear. A first grand mal seizure, for example, or a bad head injury (which might cause epilepsy) usually bring people to the doctor's office immediately. But other types of seizure symptoms are less noticeable, and it may be some time before the person sees a physician. Eventually, a fall for no apparent reason, a period of confused behavior, a sudden blackout, or some other symptom which may or may not be a sign of epilepsy—but which is a sign that something is wrong—brings the patient to the doctor's office. Or, in other cases, a routine medical checkup may lead the doctor to suspect epilepsy.

---

*Gilbert, W. S., and Sullivan, A.: "Things Are Seldom What They Seem" from *H.M.S. Pinafore*.

What Does the Doctor Do?

The examination for epilepsy begins like most other medical examinations. The doctor usually starts with the person's medical history and then goes on with a general physical checkup. Then, based on what the person has told him and what he has observed, the physician has a good idea of whether the central nervous system might be involved. If he suspects that it is, he will arrange for a neurologic examination.

The Medical History

What the patient tells the doctor is very important. It can be the way the doctor finds out whether the seizures have been recurrent and whether they are of a type that may be classified as a sign of epilepsy. It is in your own interests to be completely frank with your doctor. Detailed and accurate communication is a great help in arriving at an accurate diagnosis.

A medical history includes information about present symptoms and past illnesses. When the patient is a child, his parents or guardians will tell the doctor these things. The doctor will also ask for details about the child's birth, growth, and development. Even an adult patient often finds it helpful to have relatives present to fill in details about his childhood that he might not know or that he might have forgotten.

When he takes the medical history, the doctor also asks questions about the health of the patient's family. Some disorders do seem to run in families; and while epilepsy is usually not inherited, the family's medical history may give some clues as to what type of disorder the patient may have a tendency to develop.

If the patient has had a seizure, during the taking of the medical history the doctor will try to find out all about it. He may learn that the patient has had seizures before—perhaps without realizing it. He may learn that there have been other warning symptoms, such as a sudden tenseness or involuntary jerking or temporary numbness in an arm or leg, or twitch of the eyelids or neck, or a period of confusion—symptoms which in themselves may mean nothing, but which do point to the need for more study of the patient's condition.

With these factors in mind, the doctor is ready to give the patient a general physical examination.

The Checkup

A physical checkup is important for everybody, including people who may have epilepsy. When he examines a person, the doctor notes signs of any illness, and he may find that some condition other than epilepsy is causing the patient's symptoms.

In the case of a person with epilepsy, the checkup may provide the doctor with a clue about what caused the disorder. For example, he might notice scars from a head injury, or a laboratory test may show the presence of a blood disorder.

If the physical examination indicates that the central nervous system is involved in the patient's symptoms, the next step is a neurologic examination.

The Neurologic Examination

The goal of a neurologic examination is to find out if there is any abnormality in the brain or nervous system.

Usually a neurologist conducts the neurologic examination. A neurologist is a physician who specializes in the diagnosis and treatment of disorders of the brain and nervous system.

With the patient's permission, the doctor who did the physical examination sends the neurologist the patient's medical history and the results of the checkup and any laboratory tests (blood, urine, and so on) that have been done. The results of the physical examination and laboratory tests are referred to as the clinical findings. The neurologist reviews these clinical findings. They will be important in his final diagnosis.

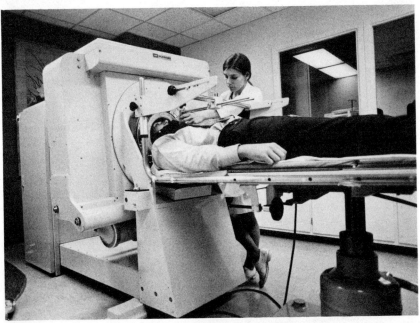

Machine used to obtain computerized axial tomography scans (CAT scans) (courtesy of The George Washington University Medical Center, Washington, D.C.)

Then the neurologist arranges for the neurologic tests. The tests are done with the latest inventions which modern technology has made possible.

One new invention is the computerized axial tomographic scan (CAT scan), which is a type of x-ray and computer combined. The CAT scan takes pictures, from various angles, of all parts of the organ under examination. Then these pictures are analyzed and put together by computer to form a three-dimensional picture which shows any abnormalities. For example, if there is a brain tumor it will show up on the CAT brain scan, and its exact location will be pinpointed. (Like an ordinary x-ray, the CAT scan takes pictures from outside the body; thus the brain is photographed through the head. See picture on page 23.)

Another major diagnostic tool is the electroencephalograph (EEG), which can help establish whether convulsions are truly epileptic in nature. The EEG examination is also painless. Electrodes, which are little flat disks or tiny needles, are placed on the surface of the scalp, between the hair. They pick

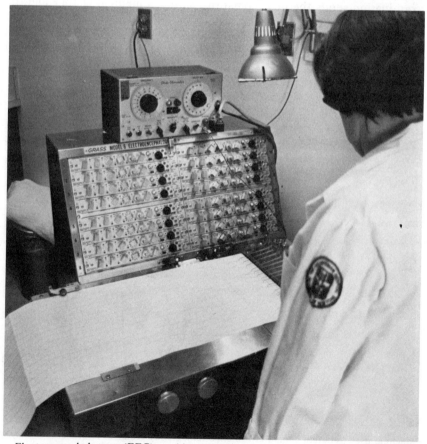

Electroencephalogram (EEG) machine (photograph furnished by Joshua Williams).

up the electrical impulses transmitted by the brain. Like a radio, the EEG machine amplifies the electrical signals. But you can't hear them; instead, they are recorded like a graph by a pen and paper attached to the machine.

The tracings that the machine makes on the paper show the wave form, voltage, and frequency of the brain waves. Sometimes the EEG shows some abnormalities. In petit mal, for example, there is usually a spike-and-wave pattern which is repeated approximately three times per second.

However, the EEG doesn't tell the whole story. In fact, in about 10 cases out of every 100, a person with epilepsy will have a normal EEG. And on the other hand there are people whose brain waves show the typical spike-and-wave pattern, but who have never had a seizure in their lives.

Therefore, doctors never depend on just one type of test. Although neurologists have now mapped the functions of most areas in the brain so well that a doctor can often tell which area is affected just by hearing a description of a seizure pattern, a diagnosis of epilepsy is never made until all test are completed and the doctor's judgment can be firmly established.

Can It Be Anything Else?

Other conditions may produce symptoms like those of epilepsy. Seizures are the predominant symptoms of epilepsy; but high fever can also cause seizures (see p. 12), and so can certain injuries, infections, and diseases.

The doctor takes all these other possibilities into consideration before he makes his diagnosis. Treatment will depend on what is causing the symptoms.

Sometimes people are apprehensive about going to the doctor. They are afraid to find out what is wrong. And so they go on suffering and worrying—often needlessly, for there may be nothing seriously wrong. Symptoms are sometimes caused by a temporary state that corrects itself right away. At other times what you think is serious is only a minor disorder that can be easily corrected with medical help. And if it does turn out that you do have what you're afraid of, isn't it better to take steps now to control it than to do nothing about it and let it get worse?

Don't try to make your own diagnosis. If you have unexplained symptoms, stop worrying and do something about it. See your doctor.

HOW CAN EPILEPSY BE TREATED?

Presiding at a now famous meeting of the Royal Medical and Chirurgical Society of London one evening in May, 1857, was Sir Charles Locock, a society doctor and Queen Victoria's personal obstetrician. The discussion that evening centered around epilepsy. Sir Charles casually remarked that he had used bromide of potassium to treat some 14 or 15 women who had epileptic seizures during their menstrual periods. The bromide treatment was a success; seizures had stopped in all but one of the patients.

Locock apparently did not realize that bromide could be used to treat all people with epilepsy. In fact, he did not even consider his discovery worth writing about. But the doctor's offhand comments signaled the discovery of a drug for which people had been searching for centuries, and the beginnings of the modern drug treatment of epilepsy.

Another doctor, Samuel Wilks, tested bromide extensively. Two years after Locock's announcement, he published his findings: bromide could successfully eliminate seizures in a large percentage of patients. From the time of Wilks's report, drugs have been the most widely used form of antiepileptic therapy.

Today, other anticonvulsant drugs have largely replaced the bromides, which, in spite of their many benefits, had some unpleasant side effects. There are many anticonvulsant drugs now available. Through medication, about half of all people with epilepsy are able to completely control their seizures, and another 25 to 30 percent achieve a marked reduction in their seizures. Thus, only about 20 percent of people with epilepsy cannot achieve significant relief with the drugs in current use.

At present, there is no cure for epilepsy. How much relief from seizures any individual can obtain depends upon his own physical reactions and the type of epilepsy he has, but drug therapy permits a growing number of people with epilepsy to live normal lives.

What Drugs Are Available Now?

Many antiepileptic drugs are now available by prescription in the United States. In deciding which drug or combination of drugs to prescribe in a given case, and the exact amount, or dosage, to use, the doctor considers the individual's general physical condition as well as the characteristics of his seizure disorder.

The major anticonvulsants that, by law, may be prescribed in this country are listed in the table on page 27.

How Do Antiepileptic Drugs Work?

Anticonvulsant drugs stop seizures from happening—that's why they are used. But how they accomplish this—how they change the seizure threshold or how they prevent electrical seizure discharge from occurring—is not fully known. We don't know the neurochemical basis for their action. We don't know why some drugs are effective against seizures while others, which seem much the same, are not. One of the goals of epilepsy research is to find out these things.

Drug research in epilepsy includes testing new preparations and

Drugs Used in the Treatment of Epilepsy

Trade Name(s)	Generic Name
Atabrine	quinacrine
Celontin	methsuximide
Clonopin*	clonazepam
Dexedrine, Benzedrine	amphetamine
Diamox	acetazolamide
Dilantin	phenytoin sodium
Gemonil	metharbital
Luminal, Stental, Eskabarb	phenobarbital
Mebaral	mephobarbital
Mesantoin	mephenytoin
Milontin	phensuximide
Mysoline	primidone
Paradione	paramethadione
Peganone	ethotoin
Phenurone	phenacemide
Tegretol*	carbamazepine
Tridione	trimethadione
Valium	diazepam
Zarontin	ethosuximide

*Tegretol and Clonopin are the newest drugs on the list; they were introduced in this country in 1974 and 1975, respectively.

investigating how anticonvulsants work. These two research areas should eventually result in medicines that are more effective and free from troublesome side effects.

Can They Tell How Much Medicine You Are Actually Getting into Your System?

The latest breakthrough in drug therapy is not a drug at all; it is a laboratory technique in which a sample of blood is taken from the patient and chemically analyzed to measure the amount of anticonvulsant drugs in the person's bloodstream.

The technique is important because it is the blood that carries the medicine to the brain, where it acts on brain cells. By monitoring how much of the drug is in the bloodstream, the doctor can tell if the person is getting the right amount of medicine. He can see when the dosage drops too low to be effective, or when drug levels become so high as to cause unpleasant or dangerous side effects. If a person is taking several medicines and having some difficulty, the doctor can tell which drug is causing the problem. Doctors used to have to figure out these things by trial and error. With blood level testing, it is much simpler to prescribe dosages that will give maximum seizure control with minimum side effects.

The first blood level testing technique, gas-liquid chromatography (GLC), was adapted for use with epilepsy in 1968. Since then, other techniques have been developed, including one called EMIT. To make these important medical tools more readily available, the Epilepsy Foundation of America has pioneered gas-liquid chromatography installations in four major clinics and is supporting the training of technicians and the establishment of quality control in laboratories performing this analysis.

Do Anticonvulsants Have Side Effects?

Anticonvulsant drugs, like all drugs, produce a variety of side effects. What these side effects are depends on the drug, how much of it is used, and the individual's reaction to that drug. One person may take quite a lot of a particular drug without any trouble, while someone else may have a strong reaction to a much smaller dose. Also, some individuals are allergic to certain drugs, and even a tiny amount can be harmful to them.

Doctors are aware that anticonvulsant drugs can have side effects, and they keep alert for signs of them. Sometimes the side effects can be corrected without too much trouble. For example, the swelling of the gums (gingival hyperplasia) sometimes produced by Dilantin can be reduced by gingivectomy, in which a dentist removes the overgrown tissue. At other times, the side effects are more bothersome.

The table on page 29 shows what side effects are sometimes produced by the anticonvulsants. The list seems long, but remember that not every person has these reactions. Many people are able to take these drugs without any unpleasantness at all.

If you have trouble with side effects, report the problem to your doctor. Remember that even a drug that you have been taking for a while may suddenly have adverse effects. This has to do with the rate with which it is absorbed into the bloodstream, and this varies as the other chemistry of the body varies.

Similarly, a drug may control seizures for a long time and then suddenly seizures break through because less anticonvulsant is being absorbed into the bloodstream. This doesn't mean that you're sicker or getting worse—everybody's body chemistry is constantly changing. Also, the number of seizures you have may not have anything to do with the underlying disorder responsible for the seizures.

So if your seizures suddenly increase, or if you start feeling ill, or sort of woozy, or unsteady on your feet—see your doctor. Remember, it is possible that any illness you have may be produced or aggravated by the drugs.

With any person for whom side effects are a problem, the doctor may decide to change to another anticonvulsant drug or to cut down on the dosage. At the same time, the doctor will want to make certain that the dosage remains high enough to control the individual's seizures. By monitoring the patient carefully with regular checkups and readings of the level of drugs in the bloodstream, the doctor can adjust the dosage to the best and most comfortable level for a particular patient.

Possible Side Effects of Drugs Used in the Treatment of Epilepsy

Drug	Some Possible Side Effects
Atabrine	Abdominal pain, diarrhea, nausea, skin discoloration, vomiting
Celontin	Dizziness, drowsiness, gastrointestinal upsets, headache, skin rash
Clonopin	Drowsiness, unsteady gait, weight gain, emotional upsets
Dexedrine	Insomnia, restlessness, weight loss
Diamox	Depression, dizziness, drowsiness, loss of appetite, numbness in arms and legs, skin rash
Dilantin	Blurred or double vision, dizziness, drowsiness, gum swelling, hair growth or loss, headache, skin rash, speech impairment, stomach upsets, unsteady gait, blood destruction
Gemonil	Drowsiness, excitability, hyperactivity, speech impairment, stomach upsets, skin rash
Luminal	Drowsiness, excitability, hyperactivity, speech impairment, stomach upsets, skin rash
Mebaral	Drowsiness, excitability, hyperactivity, speech impairment, stomach upsets, skin rash
Mesantoin	Double vision, drowsiness, skin rash, speech impairment, stomach upsets, swelling of glands, low white blood count, hepatitis
Milontin	Stomach upsets
Mysoline	Dizziness, drowsiness, headache, sexual impotence, inarticulate speech, stomach upsets, temper outbursts, skin rash
Paradione	Drowsiness, inarticulate speech, sensitivity to light, stomach upsets, blood destruction
Peganone	Depression, dizziness, double vision, drowsiness, headache, skin rash, swelling of glands
Phenurone	Depression, headaches, loss of weight, nausea, irrational behavior, stomach upsets, jaundice
Tegretol	Blurred vision, drowsiness, skin rash, stomach upsets, blood destruction
Tridione	Dizziness, headache, loss or thinning of hair, sensitivity to light, stomach upsets, swelling of joints, blood destruction
Valium	Blurred vision, dizziness, fatigue, stomach upsets, unsteady gait
Zarontin	Drowsiness, nausea, headache, sleep disturbances, stomach upsets

May a Person on Anticonvulsants Take Other Medicines?

Any mixture of drugs may produce uncomfortable, even dangerous, results. The risk of this happening is avoided when people on anticonvulsant medications check with their doctor before taking any other medicine at all, even nonprescription preparations like aspirin or antihistamines.

How about Birth Control Pills?

Many doctors advise their patients with epilepsy not to use the pill. They prescribe other methods of contraception because oral contraceptives contain hormones, estrogen and progesterone, and researchers suspect that hormones may possibly play some part in epilepsy. Another factor that researchers feel might influence the development of seizures is water retention, and in some individuals oral contraceptives cause the tissues to hold more water than usual.

Thus birth control pills may increase the risk of seizures in women with a tendency toward epilepsy, and many drug manufacturers include the following type of warning in packages of oral contraceptives: "These pills may cause some fluid retention, and conditions that might be influenced by this factor, such as epilepsy, require careful observation."

Pregnancy, Epilepsy, and Anticonvulsant Drugs

Anyone on any kind of drug should check with a doctor when having a child. During pregnancy any drug—and particularly any drug taken on a continuous basis—may be a risk to the mother or to the child.

A woman with epilepsy should discuss the matter with her neurologist before she actually becomes pregnant. The doctor will advise her about the medicines that she can safely use. If it is necessary for her to change or stop her medicine, she will be prepared to do so as soon as she becomes pregnant. In this way there will be no risk to the fetus during the important first weeks when it is developing its major form and organs.

Like all pregnant women, the woman with epilepsy can make her pregnancy safer by avoiding physical and emotional strain, getting plenty of rest, watching her diet, and immediately reporting any sudden or unusual change in her condition to her doctor.

For women with epilepsy, many doctors prescribe extra folic acid and vitamin B_{12} during pregnancy. Immediately before delivery, the obstetrician may give the mother vitamin K; immediately after delivery, he may give this vitamin to the new baby. This is because some anticonvulsants tend to cause a reduction of the blood-clotting mechanism in infants. The vitamins protect the baby from this possibility.

May a Woman on Anticonvulsants Nurse Her Baby?

Studies have shown that anticonvulsants are passed on to the child in breast milk. Therefore, whether a woman taking anticonvulsants should breastfeed her child would depend to a great extent on the amount of these drugs that she was taking. This is a question that the mother should ask the pediatric staff at the hospital where she has her baby, or her own pediatrician or family doctor.

30

May a Person on Anticonvulsants Drink?

Alcohol has different effects on different people. However, many people who take anticonvulsant drugs notice that alcoholic drinks make them feel depressed or drowsy.

Among persons with epilepsy who are not taking medication, some can tolerate moderate amounts of alcohol, while others can't. In some cases, alcohol actually causes or increases the seizures. Therefore, most doctors agree that people with epilepsy should avoid alcohol.

Can You Get Addicted to Anticonvulsants?

Recently there has been a lot of publicity about the dangers of drug abuse, and some people have become afraid of taking drugs for any reason. However, anticonvulsants are not addictive drugs, in the sense that people who take them do not develop a "drug habit," or a physical craving for the medicine.

There are important differences between taking a drug to treat an illness and abusing drugs to escape from reality. Addicts associate drugs with "highs" or pleasurable experiences that they want to repeat. Consequently, they become psychologically dependent on drugs, and this psychologic dependence remains a problem long after withdrawal and treatment have taken away the physical craving. Here addiction differs from medication; people taking anticonvulsants generally do not expect or get thrills from their medicine.

Another difference is in the amount taken. Dosages of drugs prescribed by doctors are precise and within safe limits. They're designed to give protection against oversedation on the one hand and overexcitability on the other. The dosage is seldom high enough to produce a feeling of euphoria or to mask and distort reality—which are the effects the drug abuser seeks.

There is also a difference in the reliability of the drug. Unlike many of the drugs obtained by addicts, drugs prescribed by doctors to treat an illness are chemically reliable and pure.

It is important, too, to keep in mind that most drug addicts have a psychologic problem before they start taking drugs; the addiction is actually a symptom of an underlying condition.

People who have seizures do not have this reason for taking drugs. Their motivation is simply to get relief from the seizures. Child, teenager, or adult, the epilepsy patient is taking anticonvulsant medicine only to prevent seizures and to enable him to live a normal life. In this context, anticonvulsant medications form no part of the drug abuse problem.

Do Anticonvulsants Have Any Long-Term Effects?

Some patients are worried that anticonvulsant drugs may have long-term negative effects. As noted previously, almost all of the anticonvulsant drugs may have some undesirable side effects. However, when drugs are prescribed within safe limits and are monitored by blood tests, there is no apparent long-term risk in taking them. At the same time, you must realize that these are powerful medications, and it is important to keep regular appointments for routine physical tests to ensure that everything is going well.

Doctor-Patient Teamwork

The patient and the doctor must work together as a team—a team whose goal is to fight seizures. The patient's job in this team effort is to be a good communicator. He should understand the doctor's instructions—if you're in doubt, ask!—and notice and report his reactions to the drug and the drug's effect on his seizures. The doctor's job is to consider this information and decide if any adjustments are to be made in the patient's medicine.

If a patient changes his dose himself, he makes the team effort that much harder. In such a case, the doctor finds it difficult to arrive at the best combinations and doses of drugs to control the seizures without side effects. The sudden withdrawal from medication is especially unwise because it can result in a whole flurry of seizures or in status epilepticus.

Because of his specialized training and knowledge, the doctor must be the captain of the team and the one who, taking the patient's communications into account, makes the decisions about drugs.

Does Drug Therapy Ever End?

When a person has been completely free of seizures for several years and all tests indicate that there is little chance of a seizure if he should stop taking his medicine, the doctor may decide to gradually stop the anticonvulsant drugs. For awhile after this, the patient will be carefully monitored. If seizures do not recur, the person will not be put back on medication.

Can Anticonvulsant Drugs Be Used on Animals?

Animals can get epilepsy, too. For example, epilepsy is common in dogs because of virus infections, like distemper, which can damage brain cells. Anticonvulsant drugs have been successfully used in controlling seizures in dogs. Ask your veterinarian about it.

ARE THERE ANY TREATMENTS BESIDES DRUGS?

Right now, anticonvulsant drugs are the most widely used form of treatment for epilepsy. But in a few cases, there are other methods that are used. Older techniques, including surgery and diet, and new experimental procedures, like acupuncture and biofeedback, have all been used in some cases of epilepsy.

Surgery

Although attempts at head surgery can be traced all the way back to prehistoric man, it wasn't until the end of the nineteenth century that surgical techniques advanced enough to make brain surgery effective, and that surgeons could "help the brain without mutilating it," as a leading epilepsy authority put it.*

Since the nineteenth century, brain surgery—neurosurgery, to use the technical term—has made rapid progress. Today skilled neurosurgeons successfully perform many operations that only a few years ago would have been thought impossible. The surgical treatment of epilepsy has now advanced to the point where 50 percent of carefully selected patients may be almost completely free of seizures.

There are, however, only a very limited number of patients for whom surgery is appropriate. Surgery can be undertaken only when:

1. Seizures cannot be controlled by a properly maintained regimen of anticonvulsant drugs.
2. The patient has partial (focal) epilepsy arising from a part of the brain which can be removed without causing significant physical or intellectual deficit.

Wilder Penfield, a pioneer neurosurgeon, pointed out that the doctor always considers "the best that conservative treatment can promise"† before deciding on surgery.

In epilepsy cases, brain surgery is considered only for patients whose seizures are severe and cannot be controlled by anticonvulsant drugs. There is no point in operating on a person whose symptoms are under control. Nor can brain surgery be performed unless the factor within the brain that is responsible for the seizures can be positively identified. Most importantly, brain surgery is never attempted unless it appears almost certain that the

---

*Lennox, W. G., and Lennox, M. A.: *Epilepsy and Related Disorders, vol. 2.* Little, Brown and Company, Boston, 1960, p. 892.
†Penfield, W., and Jasper, H.: *Epilepsy and the Functional Anatomy of the Human Brain.* Little, Brown and Company, Boston, 1954, p. 844.

removal of the affected brain area will help and that the person will not be harmed by the operation.

Obviously, these conditions limit the number of people with epilepsy who can be treated by surgery.

Perhaps when we know more about the mechanisms of epilepsy, surgery will have a wider role to play in its treatment. For the time being, however, drug therapy remains the treatment of choice.

Ketogenic Diets

In 1921, a new type of diet was developed that seemed to hold great promise for the treatment of epilepsy in children. This was the ketogenic diet. Within a few years, though, the ketogenic diet was largely replaced as a method of treatment by the newer anticonvulsant drugs. Generally, drugs are more effective than the ketogenic diet in controlling seizures—and they are also easier to take. But sometimes, when the drugs don't work, the diet is still used to control epilepsy.

The ketogenic diet consists of foods that are high in fat and low in carbohydrate. Confined to this regimen, the body produces "ketones," which are substances made up of acetone and diacetic acid. These substances have some anticonvulsant effect—apparently because they somehow change body chemistry.

The diet is a difficult one. A typical meal would consist, for example, of half a pound of butter and a pint of sweet cream. Fortunately, a more palatable version of the diet has recently been developed—the MCT diet.

The MCT (medium chain triglyceride) diet is another high fat, low carbohydrate diet. It is essentially a variation of the ketogenic diet, but it is easier to use because many of the fats are given in the form of a special MCT oil—and the oil can be used for cooking or mixed with other foods so that its taste is not noticeable.

Both the MCT ketogenic diet and the regular ketogenic diet should be supervised by a physician. If your doctor decides that one of them is right for your child, he will inform you about the amounts of fat to be eaten each day and will also tell you if dietary supplements, such as vitamins, are necessary.

Acupuncture

Acupuncture isn't really a new treatment; the Chinese have been using it for thousands of years. But it is only recently that Western scientists have become interested in this method of treating illnesses by inserting needles into various parts of the body.

Western research on acupuncture is still in its infancy. So far there is no evidence that this form of treatment can play a significant role in the treatment of epilepsy.

Biofeedback

We are not usually able to voluntarily control the functions of our internal organs. But it has recently been discovered that when people know what is happening inside their bodies they can sometimes learn to influence these automatic processes.

This technique is called biofeedback. In biofeedback, modern laboratory equipment and computers are used to measure physiologic processes in the body and to display them to the person in whose body they are occurring. The person can see, hear, or feel his own body working. Then he can try to influence the way it's working.

Biofeedback is being used experimentally in the treatment of epilepsy. In epilepsy, the focus is on training people to control the rhythm of their brain waves in order to avoid seizures. Researcher Maurice Sterman* believes that a brain rhythm, which he terms sensorimotor rhythm (SMR), may be able to reduce seizure activity in the brain. Dr. Sterman and his associates attempt

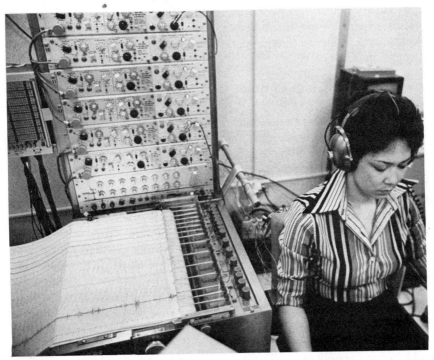

Biofeedback training (photograph furnished by Joshua Williams).

---

*Dr. Sterman is Chief of Neuropsychology Research at the Sepulveda Veterans' Administration Hospital in California.

to teach people with epilepsy to produce greater amounts of SMR in order to reduce seizures.

Biofeedback training is still very much in the experimental stage. Before this procedure can be used as a treatment for seizures, we'll have to await the outcome of research.

Can I Use My Will to Control or Stop a Seizure?

This is being researched. Behavior modification is a psychologic method that tries to change behavior by a complex system of rewards. The use of this procedure in epilepsy is based on a theory that, in some cases, we can learn to control seizures. For example, in 1973 two Massachusetts psychologists, Joseph R. Cautela and Raymond B. Flannery, reported having successfully used the techniques of behavior modification to control seizures in one epilepsy patient.*

Of course, this does not mean that behavior therapy can be used in every case of epilepsy; nor does it mean that any person with epilepsy can consciously control his own seizures. Further research will tell us how effective behavior modification can be in controlling seizures. At present, there is little evidence that people with epilepsy can control their seizures through an effort of will.

Treatments That Just Don't Work

Every type of illness and disorder has a history of many kinds of attempted remedies to cure it. In epilepsy, as in the others, many of the things that have been tried just don't work.

Sometimes a new method arouses great hopes—hopes that later prove to be unfounded. When the great Russian physiologist Ivan Pavlov announced that he had discovered a cure for epilepsy, people all over the world were enthusiastic. Unfortunately, other researchers who tried his methods found no basis for their enthusiasm. The "cure" just didn't work.

Another method that once excited great interest was GABA (gamma aminobutyric acid) treatment. It, too, was found ineffective. Indeed, the product was never even marketed.

More recently, marijuana, LSD, and other consciousness-changing drugs have been considered as possible treatments. However, there is no evidence that they help in the treatment of epilepsy, and a good deal of evidence that they hinder such treatment.

Marijuana's possibilities as an anticonvulsant are still under investigation; the results so far have been mixed. It appears to help rats and monkeys avoid

---

*Cautela, J. R. and Flannery, R. B.: *Seizures: controlling the uncontrolable.* Journal of Rehabilitation, 39:34, 1973.

seizures—but, in laboratory tests, the effect in people has so far been the exact opposite.

LSD is considered a definite hazard to people with epilepsy. In fact, in some cases it is believed to have been the trigger mechanism that actually caused the disorder in the first place.

Many other drugs, including alcohol, are harmful for people with epilepsy because they act on nerve cells. Anything that increases the hyperexcitability of neurons makes it more likely that seizures will occur.

With these drugs, as with all others, it is dangerous to be a do-it-yourselfer. If you are curious about a new method of treatment, ask your doctor about it.

WILL EPILEPSY EVER BE CURED?

In Los Angeles, California, a young man peers at a tiny nerve call through a powerful electron microscope.

In New Castle, Indiana, a doctor carefully administers a dose of a new drug to her patient.

In Bethesda, Maryland, a scientist scrutinizes the wavy line of an electroencephalograph reading.

These three people have something in common. They are all involved in

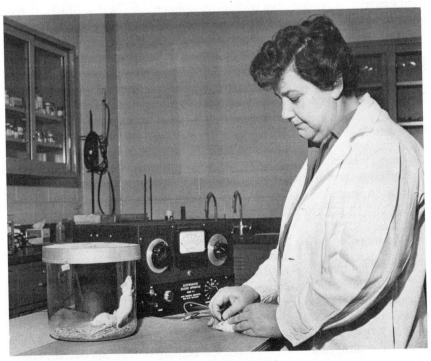

Epilepsy researcher at work.

epilepsy research. Their particular work may involve investigating the cause of epilepsy, developing new and better methods of treatment, finding ways to prevent the condition from occurring, or searching for a definitive cure.

Investigating the Brain

Our understanding of which brain processes are involved in epilepsy is still incomplete. Research to improve our knowledge of how the brain works, and then to find a method of controlling it, is progressing constantly. Discovering how the brain starts and stops seizures can help us understand the way the brain functions not only in epilepsy but also in consciousness, sleep, memory, states of mind, bodily activities, and in all other normal brain conditions.

Investigating Drugs

Neurochemists, neuropharmacologists, and other researchers hope to find more effective ways of treating epilepsy with drugs. It is possible that some day a drug will be developed that will prevent seizures in all patients; but researchers now are not concentrating on finding the one perfect drug. Instead, they are focusing on finding more effective and less toxic drugs to treat epilepsy. They are also testing antiepileptic drugs that are available elsewhere in the world but have not yet been approved for use in the United States.

Another research task is to test drugs now used in the treatment of other conditions. It is possible that some of these drugs may have anticonvulsant properties. In addition, a central thrust of basic research is to find out exactly how the drugs work on seizure mechanisms.

Investigating Surgery

A lot of research is now centered around surgery. In particular, the effects of reducing temperature are being noted. Low temperature techniques will make brain operations easier in the future; right now, these techniques are still in the early experimental stages.

Investigating Monitoring Devices

Another field for investigation is electronic controls that monitor the workings of the brain. Two types of devices are being tried: those that warn the patient when a seizure is coming on, and those that actually prevent the seizure from occurring. One instrument, developed by the McDonnell-Douglas Astronautic Company, automatically identifies the patient's EEG pattern and warns him when the electrical activity of his brain becomes the way it is before a seizure.

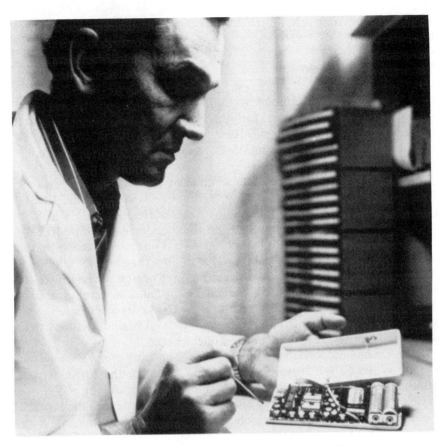

Seizure alerting device (courtesy of Dr. Frank Risch).

Other researchers, drawing upon the techniques first developed by Dr. José Delgado, are developing devices which, once they are placed within the brain, would change the electrochemical impulses that produce seizures. A device used experimentally by Dr. Irving Cooper and Dr. Sid Gilman* delivers bursts of electricity to the brain to inhibit seizures.

However, all these devices are still in the experimental stage, and their value is as yet unproved.

Testing New Treatments

New techniques and developments must be carefully tested and approved before they can be used in diagnosis or treatment. The Federal government's

---

*Dr. Cooper is Director of Neurosurgery at St. Barnabas Hospital in New York. Dr. Gilman is an H. Houston Merritt Professor of Neurology at the Neurological Institute in New York.

39

Food and Drug Administration (FDA) prohibits the use of unapproved drugs or devices.

Who Pays for Research?

Most research in the United States is done with government financial support, either in government facilities or through grants to the research facilities of universities and medical centers. That is why every time there is a cutback in government funding, the fate of research projects—a major national asset—is endangered.

The bulk of government research in epilepsy is funded by the National Institute of Neurological and Communicative Disorders and Stroke (NINCDS), a branch of the National Institutes of Health (NIH), which, in turn, is under the Department of Health, Education, and Welfare (HEW). Even though NINCDS spends millions of dollars on epilepsy research, the amount is only a fraction of what is needed to solve the problem.

NINCDS supports five special epilepsy research centers: at the University of Washington, the University of Wisconsin, the Yale University School of Medicine, the University of California, and the University of Utah. Research at these centers ranges from the general study of brain function to the development of new diagnostic and treatment methods.

NINCDS has also funded five comprehensive epilepsy program centers at the Good Samaritan Hospital in Portland, Oregon; the University of Minnesota/Mayo Clinic in Rochester, Minnesota; the University of Virginia in Charlottesville; the University of Washington in Seattle; and the Medical College of Georgia in Augusta. These centers provide multidisciplinary programs for research, treatment, evaluation, diagnosis, and handling of epilepsy-related social problems for persons with epilepsy in a defined geographic area.

Another government agency involved in epilepsy research is the Rehabilitation Services Administration (RSA), which is also under HEW. RSA sponsors research both in the United States and abroad. This agency is interested in research into the problems people with epilepsy have with employment, education, and psychologic and social adjustment.

The National Institute of Mental Health (NIMH) also funds research projects. Their investigations cover the behavioral effects of epilepsy.

Other government agencies contributing to epilepsy research include the Veterans' Administration, which operates several epilepsy centers throughout the country; the National Science Foundation, which gathers information and awards research grants; and the Department of Defense, which conducts studies on epilepsy through the Navy Bureau of Medicine and Surgery and the Army and Air Force Surgeons General.

Among private institutions, there are foundations, universities, medical schools, hospitals, and neurologic clinics throughout the country that support or conduct research into epilepsy. Drug companies also do research in this field.

The Epilepsy Foundation of America also awards grants for research projects. Through its "seed grant" programs, it has been a prime mover in starting many new pilot research projects. Seed grants are funds to get new projects started. If the projects prove promising, they subsequently can get major funding from other sources. As scientist A. B. Baker* states, "Seed grants are specifically designed to stimulate attention and encourage major funding for promising developments. When this is accomplished, research results are disseminated broadly through the Epilepsy Foundation's professional education efforts."

What Is All This Leading To?

Researchers are very optimistic about the results of their investigations. Promising avenues of research are being explored in order to learn what causes a seizure; how anticonvulsant drugs work to control seizures; what happens in the brain during a seizure; how seizures can be prevented from developing; and the many other unanswered questions which hold the key to the mystery of epilepsy.

FACTS AND FIGURES

Will a Baby Who Has a Convulsion after Running a High Fever Develop Epilepsy?

The overwhelming majority of all children who have had a febrile (fever) convulsion outgrow the tendency. Statistically, about four children out of every hundred who have a febrile convulsion develop epilepsy later on.

How Many Epilepsy Patients Can Achieve Satisfactory Seizure Control?

Approximately 80 percent of people with epilepsy can, with proper treatment and careful attention to medication schedules, achieve enough seizure control to live essentially normal lives.

---

*Dr. Baker is Head of Neurology and a Regent's Professor at the University of Minnesota. He is also past president and founder of the American Academy of Neurology, and former president of the American Neurological Association and the Epilepsy Foundation of America.

How Does a Doctor Learn of the Latest Developments in Epilepsy Research?

Research findings are published in medical and scientific journals. In addition, the American Epilepsy Society, a professional organization of scientists and physicians concerned with epilepsy, sponsors annual scientific meetings and also publishes *Epilepsia,* a scientific journal about epilepsy. Also, the Epilepsy Foundation of America publishes a *Physicians' Handbook,* and has a nationwide program of continuing education for physicians.

3

Living with Epilepsy

WHAT WILL PEOPLE THINK?

Over two thousand years ago, a doctor in Greece wrote the first book about epilepsy. The book was called *On the Sacred Disease,* and its author was Hippocrates. In the book, Hippocrates takes his fellow countrymen to task for regarding epilepsy as god-inflicted or "sacred." He states that it is a disease like any other, and, as with all diseases, its causes are to be found in the body; in this case, in the brain. Hippocrates, of course, was right; but even today, epilepsy is still regarded as being somehow more mysterious than other diseases.

The ancients regarded epilepsy as sacred because during a seizure a person often loses consciousness. The loss of control was interpreted to mean that the body had been taken over by supernatural, and probably malevolent, forces. This theory became even more popular during the Middle Ages. During this period, the belief that people's bodies could be inhabited by demons was widespread, and epilepsy, at that time called "the falling sickness," was widely attributed to demonic possession.

Such beliefs are largely responsible for the stigma traditionally attached to epilepsy. Nobody wants to associate with an "unclean" spirit.

Stigmas have a way of persisting long after their causes have disappeared. Few people today believe that epilepsy is caused by gods or demons, but some people still look upon the disorder as being somehow strange and different. This attitude can be harder for the person with epilepsy to live with than the disorder itself.

What exactly do today's people think about epilepsy? Let's see what the Gallup poll has to say about it.

The Gallup Poll

In 1949, Dr. William F. Caveness, with the help of epilepsy research pioneers William G. Lennox and H. Houston Merritt, composed a series of questions about epilepsy. The questions were used that year in a public opinion survey conducted by Dr. George Gallup of the American Institute of Public Opinion. Dr. Caveness found the results so revealing that he decided to repeat the survey to see how public attitudes change. The poll has been repeated every five years since 1949; the most recent survey was in 1974.*

The polls have shown a growing awareness of what epilepsy is, and an increase in favorable attitudes toward it. Here are the questions asked in the Gallup polls, along with a comparison of the answers given each year.

Question 1. Have you ever heard or read about the disease called "epilepsy" or convulsive seizures (fits)?

Year	Yes (%)	No (%)
1949	92	8
1954	90	10
1959	93	7
1964	95	5
1969	94	6
1974	94	6

Question 2. Would you object to having any of your children in school or at play associate with persons who sometimes had seizures (fits)?

Year	Yes (%)	No (%)	Don't know or not familiar with epilepsy (%)
1949	24	57	19
1954	17	68	15
1959	18	67	15
1964	13	77	10
1969	9	81	10
1974	5	84	11

Question 3. Do you think epilepsy is a form of insanity or not?

Year	Yes (%)	No (%)	Don't know or not familiar with epilepsy (%)
1949	13	59	28
1954	7	68	25
1959	4	74	22
1964	4	79	17
1969	4	81	15
1974	2	86	12

---

*Caveness, W. F., Merritt, H. H., and Gallup, G. H., Jr.: *A survey of public attitudes toward epilepsy in 1974 with an indication of trends over the past twenty-five years.* Epilepsia 15:523, Dec., 1974.

Question 4. What do you think is the cause of epilepsy?

Cause	1949 (%)	1959 (%)	1969 (%)	1974 (%)
Don't know	57	58	40	41
Brain, nervous system	22	27	30	26
Heredity, birth defect	12	13	19	15
Other diseases, injury	—	—	7	7
Mental or emotional	1	—	4	3
Blood disorder	2	1	3	2
Miscellaneous	7	4	2	4

Question 5. Do you think epileptics should be employed in jobs like other people?

Year	Yes (%)	No (%)	Don't know or not familiar with epilepsy (%)
1949	45	35	20
1954	60	22	18
1959	75	11	14
1964	82	9	9
1969	76	12	12
1974	81	8	11

These tables show that the trend in public attitude toward epilepsy over the past 25 years has been increasingly favorable. The poll-takers also noticed that in each of the surveys the most favorable responses came from the better educated, better employed, younger, and more urban members of the population.

The researchers themselves have some opinions as to why attitudes have improved. They believe, first, that public attitudes toward all disease have changed for the better. More specifically, they think improved medical control of seizures has contributed to a change in attitudes about epilepsy. Organizations concerned with epilepsy, such as the Epilepsy Foundation of America, have helped by educating the public about this disorder.

It seems to go like this: anticonvulsants control seizures, and public education changes attitudes.

What Do Public Service Workers Think?

It can happen this way:

On a crowded downtown street, a woman suddenly falls to the ground. A crowd gathers. Somebody calls an ambulance. When the ambulance arrives, the attendants bundle the woman onto a stretcher and take her to the hospital.

In another town, a man steps out of a restaurant and suddenly cannot remember where he is. He starts walking aimlessly down the street, moving his lips and plucking at his clothes. A policeman arrests him for drunkenness.

Both these people were having epileptic seizures. Neither of them needed any drastic sort of treatment. All they needed was someone to recognize their condition. Unfortunately, the public service workers they came in contact with didn't.

There are some ambulance attendants, policemen, firemen, airline attendants, and other people whose jobs involve serving the public who do know how to recognize a seizure and what to do about it. But there are many others who know little more about epilepsy than the public in general. It would be a community service and would save money and overburdened emergency facilities for them to learn about epilepsy.

A major effort is being made by the Epilepsy Foundation of America to educate public service personnel about epilepsy. On the local level, the Foundation conducts epilepsy training programs for policemen, firemen, emergency rescue crews, transportation personnel, and other public service workers.

The person with epilepsy can help, too. He can wear or carry medical identification that will inform public service workers that he has epilepsy. Medical identification also helps to locate the person's family, friends, or personal physician, if necessary. Emergency identification jewelry and cards are available to persons with epilepsy through membership in the Epilepsy Foundation of America.

What Do the Media Say?

The Bible mentions epilepsy. The Greeks wrote about it. Roman writers discussed Julius Caesar's attacks. Since ancient times, epilepsy has been a subject of prose and poetry, of truth and fiction.

Some writers' accounts have been purely autobiographical. Margiad Evans, for example, wrote a book about her own epilepsy. Here is what she said about one of her seizures:

The light has held patches of invisible blackness . . . one hears people ask, "What is the matter?" One cannot answer although one seems to know. One's eyes are nailed on an object or face. This rigid attitude in which one seems to be listening to a call important beyond all human matters—there is, of course, no voice. . . . The next instant I fall into nothing.*

Other writers have drawn upon their own experiences with epilepsy to describe fictional characters. In *The Idiot,* Fyodor Dostoevsky, a great Russian novelist who had epilepsy, describes an attack this way:

---

*Evans, M.: *A Ray of Darkness.* Roy, New York. 1953, p. 155.

Suddenly something seemed torn asunder before him; his soul was flooded with intense inner light. The moment lasted perhaps half a second, yet he clearly and consciously remembered the beginning, the first sound of the fearful scream which broke of itself from his breast and which he could not have checked by any effort. Then his consciousness was instantly extinguished and complete darkness followed. It was an epileptic fit.*

These are accurate descriptions of the authors' seizures, and they can be helpful to anyone who wants to learn about epilepsy. The factual acticles published in reputable newspapers and magazines, too, are usually accurate and helpful. Medical and scientific writers are, as a rule, interested in national health problems generally and are knowledgeable about epilepsy.

Unfortunately, epilepsy is not always portrayed factually. Too often, writers, filmmakers, and television personnel ignore the truth about epilepsy and distort the situation to fit their plots. This sort of literary license perpetuates mistaken notions about epilepsy.

People with epilepsy are concerned about how their disorder is portrayed because television, movies, books, and articles can all influence public opinion. And a distorted portrayal can only influence public opinion for the worse.

Changing Opinion for the Better

Good publicity, on the other hand, can help people reach a truer understanding of epilepsy. Thus, concerned people are trying to get the message across to the public.

James A. Autry, president of the board of the Epilepsy Foundation, gave these answers concerning public information when he appeared before a congressional subcommittee on public health and environment:

What segments of the audience are we trying to reach? They are many.

One, the general public, with particular emphasis on the poor and less educated;

Two, pediatricians, internists, and general practitioners whose busy schedules prevent them from having the time to discuss the disorder in depth with patients;

Three, nurses and school nurses;

Four, educators;

Five, parents and patients themselves;

Six, vocational rehabilitation specialists, employers, unions, hospitals, religious and fraternal organizations;

---

*Dostoevsky, F.: *The Idiot.* Bantam Books, New York, 1965.

Seven, insurance companies, Federal, state, and local government agencies; and

Eight, legislators.

For each of these groups the epilepsy story must be presented differently to explain how it affects their daily lives and work.*

Neal Gilliatt, vice-chairman of the Interpublic Group of Companies, one of the largest marketing and advertising agencies in the world, maintains that the task is to identify the problem, solve it from a communicator's viewpoint, then back it—to all segments of the public—with substantial media support and frequency.

But this is not an inexpensive proposition; Mr. Gilliatt estimates that at least five million dollars a year are required to sell this simple idea to the American public: epilepsy is a common disorder, and people who have it are not "different."

How Can I Change People's Attitudes?

Like many medical conditions, epilepsy is a community problem, and not just that of the person who has it. If a person is prevented from becoming a productive member of the community, he becomes instead a burden on community resources. Thus, attitudes toward epilepsy concern us all. We can each help to combat unfavorable attitudes by learning about epilepsy ourselves, and by changing our own adverse reactions and responses to it.

We can also help by getting involved in public education programs, such as those that are sponsored by the Epilepsy Foundation of America. The more you know about epilepsy the more you want to help. An educated, enlightened public can eliminate the gap between modern scientific knowledge and concepts of epilepsy and archaic views of epilepsy as a mysterious and frightening disorder.

Words Are Important, Too

Some people say that a rose by any other name is still a rose. Others believe that words play an important part in setting social attitudes; that any classification that seems to set a person apart from other people or makes him appear "different" can affect not only the way he is treated, but the way he thinks of himself—can influence his whole personality, in other words. This is particularly important during the formative years; a child is not accepted unless he is just like the other kids.

That is why, in order not to differentiate people with epilepsy from other

---

*James A. Autry, in testimony before the Congressional Subcommittee of Public Health and Environment.

people, many authorities prefer to say "a person with epilepsy"—not "an epileptic." Calling a person an epileptic tends to equate him with only one of his characteristics. A person with epilepsy may also be a teacher, an athlete, a movie star, a sports fan, a music lover, an expert cook. An individual is not exclusively any one of the things he has or the things he does; he is all of them, and more. He is, above all, a person.

HOW CAN I COPE?

What do you feel is the greatest problem you face?
　　Acceptance, self-confidence, public attitude (28.5 percent)
What do you feel is the greatest problem your child faces?
　　Stigma, social acceptance, public opinion (36 percent)

These are some of the answers received in a survey of people with epilepsy and their families.* For adults with epilepsy, public acceptance and confidence in their own abilities ranked second only to employment as a problem. For children with epilepsy, their parents believe that public acceptance is the major problem.

Self-dignity and self-worth are as important to people with epilepsy as to anyone else. A normal life is everybody's birthright. Yet people with epilepsy may find themselves faced with difficulties in many aspects of their lives—social, economic, and psychologic. The difficulties are more often caused by public opinion than by the person's medical condition. For many people, coping with public attitudes becomes a major concern.

The Problem of Rejection

Nowadays, people say that they have more favorable attitudes about epilepsy. But what people say is not always the same as how they act. Many people still act as though they believe that the person with epilepsy is somehow strange and different. Thus, a person with epilepsy may find some people rejecting him as an employee, a schoolmate, or a friend.

It is hard to live with constant rejection, and some people faced with this sort of problem have withdrawn into anger, depression, or solitude. The frustration is understandable. But these reactions don't solve anything; they just make the person feel worse, and they may lead to other problems as well.

When you are faced with rejection, it helps to understand that you are not being turned down because of any personal qualities; people are reacting to their own mistaken notions about epilepsy, not to you as an individual. They would treat any one of the millions of people with epilepsy in the same way.

---

*Gage, H. S.: *The Problems of Epilepsy as Viewed by Parents and Patients.* Epilepsy Foundation of America, Washington, D.C., 1972.

Fortunately, though, not everyone feels that way. If you're your own best friend, you'll find other friends as well. Learn to place a value on people who like you, and not on those who don't.

The Problem of Secrecy

An air of secrecy surrounds epilepsy. Some people are reluctant to report they have it—that's why statistics about the number of people with epilepsy are only estimates. Some doctors may be reluctant to diagnose it. Some people even avoid seeking medical help because they fear they may have epilepsy.

Is this secrecy justified? Will everybody be shocked if you tell them you have epilepsy?

Some people think it's all in the way you tell them. Like Nancy Swain, for example.

Nancy Swain is a Phi Theta Kappa honors student. She was "Miss Missouri-World" in 1971–72. She also has epilepsy. Here is what she has to say about telling people you have epilepsy:

Remember, it's all in the way you approach the subject. If you seem embarrassed and bashful, so will those you tell. If you discuss epilepsy with the enthusiasm of showing a friend your new shoes, your audience will be enthusiastic, too.

Ms. Swain's approach gets this message across: epilepsy is nothing to be ashamed of. That is probably the best way to tell your friends and relatives that you have epilepsy; but first you must accept your epilepsy yourself, as Ms. Swain does hers.

What about telling your acquaintances—your neighbors, your coworkers, your schoolmates? Should you tell them that you have epilepsy—even if your seizures are so well controlled that they probably would never know?

Some people feel that the subject should be wide open. They believe that epilepsy will never lose its stigma until people who have it come out of the closet and tell the world about it.

That is why people like Nancy Swain, hockey player Garry Howatt, actor John Considine, singer Ketty Lester, advertising executive Walter Howat—and many, many more—announce publicly that they have epilepsy. They hope that their speaking out will make life a little easier for other people with epilepsy.

It takes a lot of courage to speak out like this, and it doesn't always work. It can, at times, lead to misunderstandings, disappointments, and rejections. But it does take the load of secrecy and the tension off you.

Whom should you tell about your epilepsy? You must use your own good judgment. Use the method you can live with.

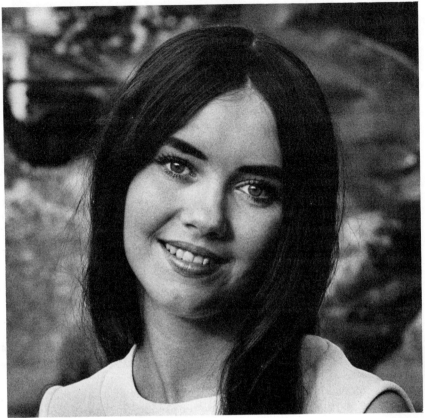

Nancy Swain.

Talking Things Over

Many people with epilepsy have found that discussing their problems makes the problems easier to live with. They have joined together into groups. Many of these groups are under the sponsorship of chapters of the Epilepsy Foundation of America. The groups are successful because the members accept each other as people, understand one another's feelings and problems, can talk things over frankly and get honest feedback, and can learn how to deal with day-by-day problems. They get strength from one another and can act collectively. They are not alone.

Professional Help

Some people who have found their emotional reactions to epilepsy hard to live with have found it helpful to talk things over with a psychologist, a psychiatrist, or a social worker. These professional people can help the person with epilepsy gain insight into his problems and to see new solutions for them. Frequently, getting in touch with his feelings gives the person a new way of coping and a new sense of hope.

Being Your Own Best Friend

People with epilepsy have also found that it helps to take an active role in their own battle. They join the fight against misunderstanding by enrolling in an epilepsy organization. Here, together with other persons with epilepsy and their families, they unite in the movement to combat prejudice against the disorder and to help all people with epilepsy lead normal lives. They are not helpless anymore; they have joined to solve those problems which require social and collective action. When one participates in this sort of action, he is no longer a passive recipient of whatever happens to be dished out; he is at last in control of his own destiny.

WILL I FIND A JOB?

It shall be an unlawful discriminatory practice for an employer, because of the age, race, creed, color, national origin, sex, or *disability* of any individual, to refuse to hire or employ or to bar or to discharge from employment such individual or to discriminate against such individual in compensation or in terms, conditions, or privileges, of employment.

New York State Executive Law
Section 292, subsection 20
(italics added)

These are the terms of a New York law that went into effect on September 1, 1974. In New Jersey, the first state to pass handicap-related anti-bias legislation, provisions specifically outlaw discrimination because of epilepsy. A number of other states also have passed such statutes.

On June 1, 1977, Section 504 of the Rehabilitation Act went into effect. The new regulations require that employers receiving Federal funds make "reasonable accommodation" for handicapped individuals.

These new rules should make it easier for handicapped people to get jobs—which, according to a 1972 survey by the Epilepsy Foundation of America, is the biggest problem for people with epilepsy. Keeping a job once their epilepsy becomes known is another problem. These problems are part of the larger problem of public attitudes. Realistically speaking, a person whose seizures are controlled can work as well and as safely as anybody else.

52

Are People with Epilepsy Good Workers?

Many researchers have made studies of how well people with epilepsy do their work. They have proved that these people are as good at their jobs as their fellow employees. In fact, some workers with epilepsy are so anxious about keeping their jobs and so eager to prove themselves that they do more than is expected of them. All in all, the job-performance ratings of people with epilepsy are equal to or better than those of their coworkers.*

Do People with Epilepsy Have Good Attendance Records?

It's hard for people with epilepsy to find work; once they find it, they don't want to lose it. They are unlikely to take time off from their jobs unless it is absolutely necessary. Their attendance records are generally excellent.

The Veterans' Administration studied the work records of 122 of its employees who had epilepsy. They found that the work performance of these employees was satisfactory, their attendance patterns normal, and that many workers had above average records.

Another researcher, S. G. Lione, studied the attendance records of people with epilepsy in industry and concluded that their "sickness and accident experience . . . is as good as, if not better than, that of the total number of employees in the working population."†

Is It Safe to Hire People with Epilepsy?

Potential employers don't have to worry about how safe it is to hire people with epilepsy. Studies have shown that they have no more accidents on the job than other workers have.

In the largest study ever made of the work records of people with epilepsy, the U. S. Department of Labor compared the employment performance of 11,000 "impaired" workers with that of 18,000 matched "unimpaired" workers.‡ They found no significant differences in performance or in accidents on the job.

Another study investigated how many job accidents were caused by epileptic seizures. Workers' Compensation records for the years 1945–1957 were examined. In this 13-year period, 8.1 out of 1,000 accident cases resulted from epileptic seizures. In the same period, 20.2 out of 1,000 accidents were

---

*Udel, M. M.: *The work performance of epileptics in industry.* Archives of Environmental Health 1:257, Sept., 1960.
†Lione, S. G.: Journal of Occupational Medicine, August, 1961.
‡*The Performance of Physically Impaired Workers in Manufacturing Industries.* U.S. Department of Labor Bulletin No. 293. U.S. Government Printing Office, Washington, D.C., 1948.

caused by coughing and sneezing.* On the basis of this study, it would seem that epilepsy is not an important factor in compensation awards. In short, people with epilepsy are not accident prone. They are safe workers.

Will My Boss's Insurance Rates Go Up?

Some potential employers say that their insurance rates will go up if they hire people with epilepsy. This is believed to be only an excuse, because insurance rates—according to official company statements—are determined by the claim record of the company, not by the medical conditions of individual employees. Insurance companies say that they do not tell employers whom to hire, and that people with epilepsy are eligible to participate in company health plans just like anyone else.

Government insurance programs work on the same principle. In each state, employers are required to carry Workers' Compensation insurance. If an employee is injured on the job, he is paid damages from the state's Workers' Compensation fund. Compensation and insurance rates vary from state to state; but they are always determined by the state government, not by the employer. In determining the rates employers have to pay, the state considers how hazardous each type of business is, and how many accidents have occurred there in the past. The number of handicapped people employed and the physical condition of the employees are not considered.

In fact, epilepsy causes so few accidents that it isn't mentioned as a separate category even for statistical purposes, a survey of state industrial accident boards and Workers' Compensation commissions throughout the country revealed.

Some state-run insurance programs have been designed especially to encourage employers to hire handicapped workers. Forty-six states and the District of Columbia have Second Injury funds. This means that if a person who is already disabled has an accident on the job, he is paid for any further disability from this state fund; his employer does not have to pay. There are only two states that specifically mention epilepsy in the provisions for the Second Injury fund. Nevertheless, most other states also consider epilepsy one of the eligible disabilities.

One thing to watch: Usually neither an employer nor a worker can get the Second Injury benefits unless the employer knows of the worker's epilepsy beforehand.

What Should I Say in the Application?

People with epilepsy are efficient, reliable, and safe workers. The problem is to convince a prospective employer of these facts.

---

*Commission on Neurological Disorders in Industry, Council on Industrial Health, American Medical Association. *Abstract*. Epilepsy News 8:1, 1961.

Or should you even try? Some researchers have concluded that many employers who know the facts won't hire people with epilepsy anyway—simply because of their own prejudices against them.*

For this reason, some people don't tell prospective employers about their epilepsy. Even if the application form specifically asks this question, they answer no.

However, this creates its own problems. If he gets the job, the person who has concealed epilepsy will constantly be worried that the truth will come out; because, if it does, the company may fire the worker on the grounds that he lied on the job application.

People with epilepsy are caught in a double bind. If they tell the truth, they may not be hired; if they tell a lie, they may be fired.

Many people have decided that it is better to tell the truth than to worry about the secret being discovered. They come to job interviews armed with proof about their abilities, statistics about how well people with epilepsy do on the job, and a note from their doctor saying that their seizures are controlled, that their medical condition will not affect their work, and that they are safe workers. In many cases, these people are able to convince a prospective employer and are hired.

What If I'm Fired Without Cause?

Many people with epilepsy are fired or forced to resign or retire from their jobs once their epilepsy is discovered. Sometimes workers are dismissed after they have a seizure on the job. This doesn't really make sense. If the business is such that a seizure is a safety risk—OK. But if a seizure isn't a safety risk to the person himself, his coworkers, or the company's equipment, it shouldn't be a reason for dismissing a good worker. The real reason is probably emotional; the employer doesn't understand epilepsy, thinks there's something bad about it, and is upset by the seizure.

In the states that now outlaw discrimination against people with disabilities, including epilepsy, the employee who is dismissed because of his disorder has legal grounds for getting his job back, unless the employer can show that the handicap directly related to his ability to perform his job safely. If you live in a state with such a law and you have been illegally dismissed, get in touch with your state's commission on human rights, your lawyer, or your legal aid society to find out what to do.

In addition, if you are fired because of epilepsy—or told that you cannot be hired because you have epilepsy—you may have cause for legal action under Section 503 of the Federal Vocational Rehabilitation Act of 1973. With this act, Congress told all businesses which do work amounting to more than

---

*Sands, H., and Zalkind, S. S.: *Effects of an education campaign to change employer attitudes toward hiring epileptics.* Epilepsia 13:87, Jan., 1972.

$2,500 a year for Federal or state governments that they could not discriminate against employees or potential employees on the basis of physical handicaps—and that includes epilepsy.

Today most large companies, and many small ones as well, have contracts to sell goods and services to the government; so it may be worthwhile to check with the Employment and Training Administration of the Department of Labor if you think your rights under this provision have been violated. Remember, you must prove that you are well qualified for the position—not always an easy thing to do, since none of the laws define qualifications—and that the only reason you have been rejected is because of epilepsy.

If none of these provisions apply to your job, or if legal action is a step you hesitate to take, there are some other things you can try first. Sometimes it works if you get someone else to speak to your employer on your behalf. The advocate might be your doctor or a counselor from the handicap division of the state employment agency or from the Division of Vocational Rehabilitation or from your local Epilepsy Foundation chapter. Your advocate could present the facts about your condition and explain them to your boss. He might be able to persuade him that is it in his best interests to rehire you.

Is There Any Job I Shouldn't Try?

Doctor, lawyer, merchant, chief—people with epilepsy are employed in just about every kind of job there is. Like other people, they choose their careers on the basis of their abilities, capabilities, and interests.

However, the person with epilepsy must also take into account how well his seizures are controlled, how reliable the aura is as a warning that a seizure is coming on, the kind of seizure he has, the safety risks of the job he is thinking about, and how all these factors interrelate.

Consider your own situation realistically, and choose a job that is consistent with your own safety and that of your coworkers.

What about Military Service?

One career that is still barred to people with epilepsy—regardless of their seizure control—is the military. Army Regulation 40-501 states:

Paroxysmal convulsive disorders, disturbances of consciousness, all forms of psychomotor or temporal lobe epilepsy or history thereof except for seizures associated with toxic states or fever during childhood up to the age of five are cause for rejection for appointment, enlistment, or induction.

Since physical standards for joining any branch of the service are those set forth in Army Regulation 40-501, this regulation applies to all the armed services.

56

This rule presumably exists because military recruits must be physically fit to serve in an unrestricted capacity anywhere in the world, including isolated posts and stations where doctors and medicines are not readily available—although there would seem to be no reason why people with epilepsy couldn't be sent to posts where they were accessible. It would be truly a public service for the military to lead the way in this fashion.

There are some people with epilepsy in the armed services, though; they developed epilepsy after they joined. When a person develops epilepsy while he is in the service, his future career depends on the conditions that precipitated the epilepsy. If he had no previous history of the disorder and he developed epilepsy within four months after he got in, he is usually discharged "under honorable conditions." If the epilepsy begins or is discovered after the fourth month, the service has the option of retaining or of discharging the person; sometimes he may be kept on as a volunteer. In evaluating such a case, the authorities consider whether the condition can be controlled by standard anticonvulsant drugs and whether the person needs clinical and laboratory tests frequently. They also consider the length of time the person has already served and how much they need his particular military occupational specialty. When a person with epilepsy is kept on, the service usually imposes certain conditions. Generally, the person is given only assignments and duties where a sudden loss of consciousness would not be dangerous to himself or to others.

Who Can Help Me Find a Job?

There are groups that specialize in helping handicapped people get jobs. The major organizations doing this type of work are the state Division of Vocational Rehabilitation, some state employment services, and the voluntary health organizations.

The Division of Vocational Rehabilitation (DVR) is a state-Federal agency with district offices in every state and territory of the nation. DVR helps anyone with a physical and/or emotional disability who is not gainfully employed, or who is working below his potential. According to recent legislation, priority for DVR services must go to the most severely disabled; also according to these laws, epilepsy is included as a severely disabling condition and is a current priority.

The range of services offered by DVR is wide: medical and psychologic examinations and treatment, vocational testing and counseling, vocational training, and job placement in industry or, where called for, sheltered workshops.

To get in touch with DVR, contact the State Commission of Vocational Rehabilitation in your state capital.

Another resource is your state employment service. Many state employment services have counselors especially assigned to job placement with the handicapped. Ask the state employment office in your area whether they provide such a service.

The state and local chapters of the Epilepsy Foundation of America can also help to find jobs for people with epilepsy.

CAN I HAVE A NORMAL FAMILY LIFE?

Once upon a time—not so long ago, either—people with epilepsy were advised not to marry; and in many states they were even prevented from marrying by law. But now it is known that there is no reason for people with epilepsy not to marry. Legal restrictions have been removed. There is nothing to prevent people with epilepsy from having a normal and satisfying family life—but epilepsy does present an additional challenge.

Marriage Laws

The laws that prevented people with epilepsy from marrying were based on mistaken notions about heredity and on the belief that people with epilepsy would end up in an institution. When modern understanding of epilepsy reached the lawmakers, the antimarriage laws began to disappear. The last such law was repealed in 1969, and now people with epilepsy can legally be married anywhere in the United States.

Should I Tell My Partner about My Epilepsy?

If your partner is a casual date and still a stranger, use your own judgment about telling him or her of your epilepsy, just as you would about other personal things. But if your partner is your husband or wife—or someone with whom you've formed a significant relationship—then tell them. Openness is an essential condition for a significant, trusting relationship. Hiding important information about yourself leads to mistrust and resentment. It can even be grounds for annulment or divorce.

Tell your partner, and free yourself from the fear that he or she will find out.

Will Epilepsy Interfere with My Sex Life?

Epilepsy has no effect on a person's physical ability to have sexual intercourse. The one exception to this rule is that some men taking the anticonvulsant drug Mysoline may become temporarily impotent. This symptom disappears when the men become accustomed to the drug or are switched to other medications.

The desire for sexual intercourse often depends on one's mood. If a person is feeling tired, or depressed, he or she just may not feel like having intercourse. If this feeling persists, the person should see their doctor.

58

Tiredness and depression may be side effects of anticonvulsant drugs—and if they are, the doctor may be able to adjust the dosage to get rid of these effects. If something else is causing these troublesome feelings, the doctor may be able to suggest some other remedy.

Should I Have Children?

Epilepsy is not generally passed from parent to child; but there is, it is true, a slightly higher chance that a child with one parent with epilepsy will develop the condition, and the chance increases somewhat if both parents have epilepsy. A genetic counselor can tell you what the odds for your child are.

The degree to which epilepsy can now be treated should also be a factor in a couple's decision on whether or not to have a child.

Often the most important question may be: Can you cope with epilepsy sufficiently to deal with your children and their reactions to your seizures?

Can a Person with Epilepsy Be a Good Parent?

Having children is an additional challenge for people with epilepsy. The challenge varies with the kind and frequency of the seizure and the age of the child.

Parents with epilepsy have realistic concerns about their children: Will a mother drop her infant during a seizure? (Not if the seizures are well controlled, or if she has warning symptoms in advance, or if there is somebody else standing by to take care of the child in an emergency.) Will a father frighten his six-year-old if he has a seizure? (Not if the parents have been open with the child and have explained to him, in simple terms, what to expect.) Will the teenager's date become embarrassed if he witnesses a parent's seizure? (Not if the date has been prepared for it and the family is unembarrassed.)

All these concerns can be dealt with if both parents cooperate and are open and honest and understanding. Remember, it is the parents who serve as models for their children and help determine their attitudes.

CAN I BE ACTIVE?

When a New Jersey court decided in his favor recently, skydiver John Langenbach was jubilant. Mr. Langenbach had been barred from jumping at a local airfield because of his epilepsy. Basing his case on New Jersey's antidiscrimination law, Mr. Langenbach filed a complaint with the state's Division on Civil Rights. Because his seizures are reliably controlled, the court ordered the airfield to allow the skydiver to use its facilities.

Mr. Langenbach is just one of many athletes who have refused to let

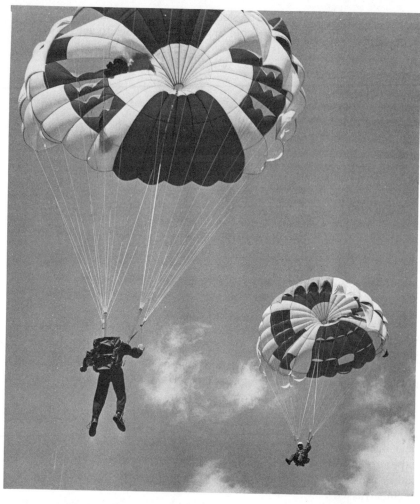

Skydivers (Harold M. Lambert Studios, Inc., Philadelphia, Pa.).

epilepsy ground them. Not all of them are skydivers. Some are hockey players—like the New York Islanders' Garry Howatt. Some are runners—like British marathon star Alan Blinston. Some are baseball players—like the New York Yankees' great Tony Lazzeri.

These sports stars prove that epilepsy needn't stop you from living an active life.

Is Exercise Good for Me?

Exercise is good for everybody, and the person with epilepsy is no exception. In fact, there is some evidence that exercise may be especially

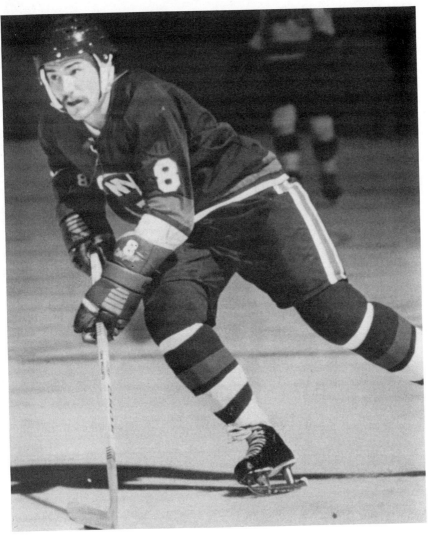

Garry Howatt (*Focus on Sports* photograph by Jerry Wacther).

good for people with epilepsy. In a University of Nebraska study supported by a research grant from the Epilepsy Foundation of America, Dr. Kenneth Rose and his research team are investigating the effects of exercise on epilepsy. Early findings suggest that exercise may temporarily ward off seizures.

If you aren't used to exercise, ask your doctor about it. He will probably advise you to start gradually. Walking is a good activity to begin with. So are bowling and golf.

What About Swimming?

Most people with epilepsy may go swimming—*if* their seizures are under control, and *if* they follow simple safety precautions. Even well-controlled people with epilepsy may have an occasional seizure—and since seizures usually start with a quick inhalation of breath, if the seizure takes place in the water, a lot of water is sucked in. Of course, this is dangerous. So be sure that someone close by keeps a watch on you when you go swimming.

Here are some rules for safe swimming for people with epilepsy:

Ask your doctor about swimming, and follow his advice.

Don't ever swim alone, or in areas far from help.

Tell school authorities, lifeguards, swimming teachers, and camp counselors if you have epilepsy and want to swim. It's not fair to them if you don't, and it could be fatal to you.

Don't swim if you have forgotten to take your medication at the time it was scheduled; don't swim if you're not taking your prescribed medicine regularly.

If a child who has seizures is playing near the water, make sure that he is wearing a lightweight life jacket or a small plastic foam flotation device, and that there is someone watching him.

For people whose seizures are less well controlled, here's more advice:

Swim only with a buddy who knows about your condition.

Wear a bright-colored bathing cap for quick visibility.

An inflatable belt of the type used by divers is a good idea—your buddy can pull the rope to inflate the belt if necessary.

Consider that seizures and swimming do pose a hazard, and that you should perhaps wait until you have better control before you go swimming.

What About Diving? Scuba Diving? Snorkeling?

All the varieties of diving are hazardous for people whose seizures are not perfectly—and we mean 100 percent!—controlled. Imagine the dangers of an underwater blackout. Even if you feel great today, it's no guarantee against having a seizure. Only if you are certain that your seizures are reliably controlled—if you have had no seizures for five years—should you consider taking part in these sports. However, first speak to your doctor.

Play it safe. Use the buddy system, and alert your companion that, although the possibility is remote, you may have a seizure. Tell your buddy that if anything peculiar seems to be happening to you, he is to pull you up at once.

What About Riding a Bicycle?

Bicycle riding is fun, but it brings with it the risk of traffic accidents. For children and adults with good seizure control, this risk is no greater than for people who don't have epilepsy. When control is less reliable, bicycle riding should be confined to safe places such as parks and special bicycle paths. These are intelligent and reasonable precautions, not unfair restrictions.

What About Riding a Motorcycle?

Motorcycling demands complete alertness and muscular control. Only those people whose seizures are completely controlled should take part in it. In fact, driver's license laws in your state will determine whether or not you may have an operator's license.

What About Horseback Riding?

People whose seizures are under control may go horseback riding. But it is best not to ride alone. And to avoid the risk of head injury in case of a fall, stable owners advise all riders—with or without epilepsy—to wear hard hats.

What About Climbing?

Doctors advise people who are still having seizures to avoid climbing—and this includes mountain climbing, tree climbing, and working on ladders.* The danger of a loss of consciousness when a person is perched above the ground is obvious. The degree and reliability of seizure control will determine the risk.

What About Contact Sports?

For a long time doctors felt that people with epilepsy should not take part in body contact sports, such as boxing, football, soccer, and rugby. However, medical authorities have now decided that, if control is good and the individual wants very much to take part in them, these sports should not be forbidden to people with epilepsy.

In a 1974 statement, the American Medical Association (AMA) declared, "There is ample evidence to show that patients will not be affected adversely by indulging in any sport, including football, provided the normal safeguards for sports participation are followed, including adequate head protection."†

*Livingston, S.: *Comprehensive Management of Epilepsy in Infancy, Childhood and Adolescence.* Charles C Thomas, Springfield, Ill., 1972, p. 145.

†Corbitt, R. W.: *Epileptics and contact sports.* Editorial. Journal of the American Medical Association 229:820, August 12, 1974.

While the AMA no longer rules out participation in rough-and-tumble activities, it still prefers the choice of noncontact sports for people with epilepsy.

My Hobby Is . . .

Parties, dancing, movies, television, the theater, the opera—you name it. People with epilepsy take part in the same kinds of recreational activities that everybody else does. Like everyone else, the person with epilepsy can, and should, live a full and active life. As a matter of fact, this is essential for good adjustment!

Don't be dull and dreary and blame it all on epilepsy. If you become active in all spheres of living, you'll find yourself coping as successfully with epilepsy as with everything else.

WHAT ARE MY RIGHTS?

It seems obvious that a person with epilepsy should have the same rights guaranteed by the United States Constitution as anybody else. Yet, in actual fact, many of the millions of Americans with epilepsy are often discriminated against. The discrimination continues, although most of the laws once directed against people with epilepsy have now been repealed. To ensure the rights of people with epilepsy, we need new laws—laws that expressly forbid discrimination.

Laws that Discriminate

Marriage, immigration, driving—at one time people with epilepsy were legally discriminated against in all these areas. Now the law has finally caught up with modern thinking, and most of the prohibitions have been removed.

The last state statute forbidding the marriage of people with epilepsy was repealed in 1969 (the state was West Virginia). Immigration laws were changed a few years earlier. Before 1965, people with epilepsy were barred from immigrating to the United States. In 1965, the Federal Immigration and Nationality Act was revised, and people with epilepsy were no longer excluded from the country.

Some discriminatory laws still exist. There are a few states where an adoption can be legally annulled if the adopted child develops epilepsy, and several states with laws whereby people with epilepsy can be sterilized. Although these laws are almost never enforced nowadays, the mere fact that they exist can foster mistaken notions of the nature of epilepsy.

Laws concerning driving used to be discriminatory; but now they try to take into account that driving is a necessity of daily living and that people with epilepsy should be allowed to drive, as long as public and individual safety are respected.

Driving Laws

Driving a car is always a risky business. Each year hundreds of thousands of people are injured in automobile accidents. Obviously, a person who might suddenly become unconscious at the wheel increases the risk. However, people whose seizures are completely controlled, whose seizures occur only during sleep, or who have sufficient and reliable enough warning time before a seizure to enable them to pull over to the side of the road and stop the car are not undue safety risks.

Every state now grants driver's licenses to people with epilepsy who can satisfy officials that they have achieved control of the disorder and will be safe drivers.

In most states, a certificate from a doctor stating that a person with epilepsy has had seizure control for a specified time period—usually a year or two—is enough to assure state officials that the person can operate a car safely (provided, of course, that he can also pass the usual driving and vision tests).* Some states also require people with epilepsy to undergo physical examinations, including electroencephalography. In these states, licenses must be frequently renewed as a means of monitoring the person's degree of control.

I Can't Get a License: What Can I Use as Identification?

In our society, driver's licenses are so frequently used as a means of identification that the person who cannot get one often has trouble cashing checks, registering at hotels, and coping with other situations where he has to prove his identity.

If you need identification, check with your state. Some states do issue ID cards—sometimes through the state liquor authority or department of motor vehicles.

An excellent means of identification is a passport. Although we rarely think of using a passport within the United States, it is always acceptable ID. To find out how to get a passport, phone the passport agency; it is listed in the phone book under United States Government, State Department.

---

*Schwade, E.: *Medical certification of seizure control.* In Wright, G. N. Gibbs, F. A., and Linde, S. M. (eds.): *Total Rehabilitation of Epileptics—Gateway to Employment.* Office of Vacational Rehabilitation, Department of Health, Education, and Welfare, Washington, D.C., 1963, p. 22.

I Got a License: Can I Get Car Insurance?

Automobile insurance laws vary from state to state. In general, there are two sources of auto insurance: (1) private insurance companies and (2) state assigned-risk plans.

Often, people with epilepsy can't get regular automobile insurance from private companies. That's because insurance underwriters tend to assume—even without evidence—that people with epilepsy have a higher than average chance of being involved in automobile accidents. Even when people with epilepsy can get private insurance, they usually have to pay higher than average premiums.

Some people, however, can use the other source of insurance. If the private companies turn down a person's application for car insurance, he can apply for coverage through the state's assigned-risk plan. In certain states, however, people with epilepsy are not eligible for the state coverage.

If you are having trouble getting automobile insurance, consult your local or state insurance commissioner for information and assistance.

What About Life Insurance?

Auto insurance isn't the only problem. Life and health insurance can cause trouble, too.

In theory, when a person with epilepsy applies for life or health insurance his application should be treated according to the same actuarial standards that apply to other people. The insurance company should base its acceptance or refusal as well as its rates on the chances of having to pay a claim to the applicant.

Unfortunately, many insurance companies merely assume that the person with epilepsy is a poor risk. Where insurance is concerned, when a person is classified as a poor risk he either has to pay more for his policy or must deal with an insurance company that specializes in substandard policies that lack important protection.

Fortunately, for the first time in the history of this country, a national group life insurance plan has been designed by the Epilepsy Foundation of America specifically to include people with epilepsy.

The insurance is provided by a well-known company, the Government Employees Life Insurance Company, an affiliate of GEICO. It provides up to $25,000 of term insurance at low group rates and is offered to members of the Epilepsy Foundation and their families, including people with epilepsy and those without epilepsy.

Dr. Adolph L. Sahs, a distinguished neurologist and chairman of the board of the Epilepsy Foundation, has called the development "a major service to people with epilepsy." He says, "One of the biggest problems faced by people with epilepsy has been the inability to secure basic life insurance coverage. Modern treatments have made it possible for many more people with epilepsy to lead normal, productive lives, and this is recognized in this insurance program and its low premium rates."

Information about the EFA Group Life Plan and rates can be obtained from your local chapter of the Epilepsy Foundation of America.

What About Health Insurance?

Health insurance is even harder to get from private companies than life insurance, because the insurance companies assume that people with epilepsy will need a lot of medical treatment. Sometimes the person with epilepsy has to settle for a policy that excludes payments for any treatment connected with epilepsy, and even then, premiums may be unusually high.

In some states, such discrimination is illegal. But in most states, the best solution to the insurance dilemma is for the person with epilepsy to enroll in a group insurance plan if he has the chance to do so. In group insurance plans, the premiums are usually lower. More important, coverage is often automatic for all members of the group—the state of any individual's health doesn't matter.

What About Social Security?

Some people with epilepsy are eligible for Social Security benefits. Under Federal law, Social Security payments may be made to disabled people, and the definition of a disability includes epilepsy if seizures are not controlled.

In a recent letter to the Epilepsy Foundation, the Social Security Administration stated:

To meet the disability requirement, an individual must have a medically determinable impairment that has prevented or is expected to prevent him from engaging in his usual work activity or any other substantial gainful work for a continuous period of at least 12 months. Since the social security law provides that the definition of disability applies to all medically determinable conditions, disability claims from persons with epilepsy are given the same consideration as those from other individuals.

Generally, an individual with epilepsy will meet the disability requirement if he has major motor seizures (loss of consciousness and convulsions) substantiated by clinical findings and occurring more frequently than once a month in spite of prescribed treatment. He will also usually qualify if he has minor motor seizures (alteration of awareness or loss of consciousness) substantiated by clinical findings and occurring more frequently than once a week in spite of prescribed treatment. Where adequate seizure control is obtained only with unusually large doses of medication, consideration is given to any impairment resulting from the side effects of this medication. Consideration is also given to impairment-related work restrictions, such as avoiding work around moving machinery.

An individual with epilepsy not as severe as described above might still qualify for benefits if he has an additional impairment or if his condition, considering his age, education, and work experience, nonetheless prevents him from engaging in substantial gainful activity.*

For information about how to apply for Social Security, contact your local Social Security office.

. . . And Medicare?

People who receive Social Security disability benefits are also eligible for Medicare's free hospital benefits. In 1977, the benefits include all hospital costs over $124 for the first sixty days in hospital, and all costs over $31 up to ninety days.

Laws Against Discrimination

New York and New Jersey's antidiscrimination amendments have already been mentioned (page 52) as laws designed to protect people with a physical disability. These laws make it illegal to discriminate against handicapped people in employment and in other areas. New York's law would cover people with epilepsy in its general definition of disabled people; New Jersey's Law Against Discrimination is one of the few antidiscrimination laws in the nation to specifically mention epilepsy.

Other states, too, have passed or are considering laws forbidding discrimination against the disabled. An increasing number of legislators recognize that people with epilepsy are being treated unfairly. The laws that have already been passed could well serve as models for other states to legally protect the rights and privileges of those with epilepsy, and to offer them the same safeguards afforded other people who are discriminated against. Getting these laws enforced and observed is an important step in getting rid of employment discrimination—and all discrimination.

If You Are Discriminated Against

The remedy for discrimination varies according to what type of discrimination you have suffered and whether or not this type of discrimination is illegal in your state.

---

*Samuel E. Clouch, Acting Director, Bureau of Disability Insurance, Social Security Administration, letter to the Epilepsy Foundation of America, June 5, 1975.

A good place to call for information about the measures you can take is your local chapter of the Epilepsy Foundation of America.

Other good sources of help are the American Civil Liberties Union, the state attorney general, and your local legal aid office. In Massachussetts there is also a legal defender whom you can contact.

If your state has an antidiscrimination law, the state's Division of Human Rights can give you information about what legal action to take.

Your state senator or representative may also be of help. Many elected officials will fight cases of blatant discrimination against individuals.

For additional pointers, see the section on employment discrimination, pages 55 and 56.

Advocacy and the Law

Advocacy means to publicly promote a cause. In the epilepsy movement, advocacy means helping people with epilepsy by representing their rights to legislators, to employers, to service agencies, and to the public at large.

Health organizations have recently been increasing their advocacy activities. They know that advocacy is one way to provide better service to those with epilepsy and other handicapping conditions.

One organization whose activities center around advocacy is the National Center for Law and the Handicapped, Inc., 1235 North Eddy Street, South Bend, Indiana. The National Center is supported by a grant from the United States Department of Health, Education, and Welfare, Its purpose is to provide up-to-date information about social and legal actions conducted throughout the United States on behalf of handicapped persons.

People with epilepsy can become their own advocates by joining together to make their needs known to their elected representatives. With other members of the epilepsy movement, they can support legislators who support them. This sort of advocacy will eventually lead to increased opportunities for employment and education, improved state and Federal services, and new statutes to finally bring to an end discrimination against people with epilepsy.

FACTS AND FIGURES

How Many People Have Trouble Getting a Job Because of Epilepsy?

Over 42 percent of the people answering a 1972 Epilepsy Foundation of America questionnaire said that they had had problems in getting a job.

What Laws Would Most People with Epilepsy Like to See Passed?

A large number of people with epilepsy (40.7 percent) believe that the laws that would help them most would be laws against discrimination in hiring.

4

The Child with Epilepsy

HOW WILL EPILEPSY AFFECT MY CHILD?

Even when seizures are well controlled, it is true that epilepsy is bound to affect a child's life. There are the daily doses of medication, the more than usual visits to the doctor—and the self-questionings and self-doubts that arise in the minds of child and parents alike.

These are serious problems. But they can be overcome. A letter recently received by the Epilepsy Foundation of America makes this clear:

Dear Neighbor,

There is a little guy living at my house that I would like you to know about. This little guy is only ten years old and he's all boy. He does fairly well in school, having the usual problems with his teachers, but the reasons for these problems are a little unusual.

But don't get me wrong—he is smart as a whip and could be a straight "A" student if he applied himself. This little guy is a pretty good musician, too—he loves to sing, sings pretty loud, right on pitch I might add, and can even accompany himself on a ukulele.

He is stumbling around with trying to learn the clarinet, and his teacher says that he could be great if, again, he would apply himself and practice.

He's been playing organized soccer for a couple of years now and really does a fine job for the team. Nothing flashy or extraordinary, but usually plays his assigned position very well.

He's been "Little Leaguing" it for a couple of years and when he learns to hit, there will be a lot of coaches wanting him on their team. He doesn't play football now and it is very doubtful if he ever will, but you will understand why as you read along.

Neighbor, if you haven't already, I hope that you have the opportunity

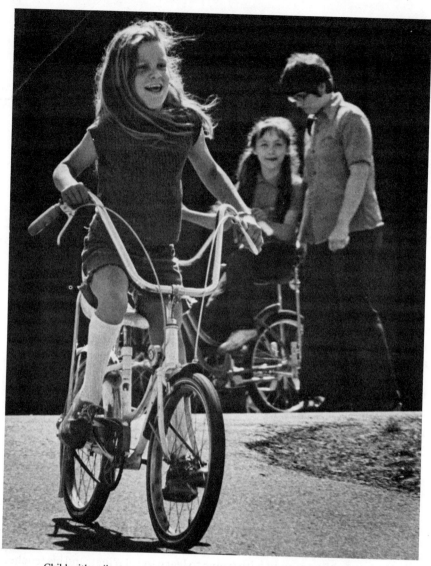

Child with epilepsy at play (*Statesman Journal* photograph by Dan Poush).

some day to meet this little guy. I am very proud of him and I should be, because he is my son. Perhaps you have a son or know several boys about this age, but there is probably a big difference between them and the one at my house.

You see, neighbor—my little guy has epilepsy.

The letter is signed, "A Very Proud Father."

What Should I Tell My Child?

A little girl was reading a rather lengthy book about penguins. Someone asked her how she liked it. "Oh," replied the little girl, "it told me more about penguins than I wanted to know."

Don't tell your child more about epilepsy than he is ready to know. If your child is very young, he will probably be satisfied with this sort of explanation: "The doctor says you have to take your medicine every day for these spells."

With an older child, the disorder can—and should—be discussed more thoroughly; but again, the discussion should go only as far as the child desires and is able to understand. Do give the child honest answers to his questions; don't raise issues that haven't occurred to him yet.

Don't stress the negative. It is always better to put the emphasis on the fact that the medicine helps the child stay well, not on the fact that he has an illness. It is better to stress the things the child can do, not those he can't.

Be open to the child's needs. Let him express his negative feelings and experiences. And let him know that you understand.

How Can I Be Sure that My Child Takes His Medicine?

When children are very small, it is relatively easy for parents to see that they get their medicine. But as the child gets older, the job may get harder; for, as part of learning responsibility and independence, the responsibility for taking the anticonvulsant drugs should be gradually transferred to the child. A child needs responsibilities like this; they help him grow into an independent and self-confident adult. Care of oneself is an important lesson for every child to learn.

Parents may feel uneasy, at first, about giving the child this responsibility. But the child will usually justify his parents' trust if he is confident of their faith in him and if he realizes the importance of the task.

It also helps the child remember if a regular schedule is set for taking medicine. One way to do this is to make it part of another daily routine. The child can take his pills at mealtimes, for example, or just before he brushes his teeth, or at bedtime—or ask your doctor for a good time schedule so that the child can develop the habit of taking his medicine with 100 percent reliability.

Can I Leave My Child with a Babysitter?

When you want to go out, it is a good idea to leave your child with a babysitter. It shows that you aren't afraid—a good example to set and another step toward your child's independence. It is good for the child to realize that his parents don't have to stay with him all the time.

A quiet talk with the babysitter on what to do if the child has a seizure is a good idea. Letting the babysitter know what to expect will remove any fears or uneasiness that he may have.

Does My Child Need Extra Rest?

The child with epilepsy needs the same amount of rest as other children his age—no more, and no less. Once he is past babyhood, he should not be forced to take regular rest periods or a daily nap. This sort of treatment will only make the child feel like an invalid.

Instead of being forced to rest, the child with epilepsy should be encouraged to play with other children, take part in sports, and live as active a life as he can. Fresh air and exercise are good for kids—and that includes kids with epilepsy.

Is It OK to Discipline My Child?

Children need discipline. Not harsh, overly strict discipline—but a firm, warm expectation that they will live up to certain rules and respect certain limits. This kind of discipline gives children a feeling of security and personal controls.

Sometimes parents are afraid that their child will have a seizure if he doesn't get his own way. But he won't. And if he is allowed to behave in ways that he wouldn't get away with if he didn't have epilepsy, he soon understands that he is getting special treatment. Also, he begins to feel different from other children—perhaps inferior to them. Or he may try to adjust by using the ailment as an excuse for not taking part in normal activities.

The best way to treat a child with epilepsy is, as nearly as possible, the way you treat other children. With discipline, that means using the same methods you use for the rest of your family.

What About My Other Children?

Traditionally, there's a lot of rivalry between brothers and sisters, and the rivalry becomes stronger if one of the children is given special treatment. Other children in the family resent the child whom they think their parents are favoring, and they resent their parents for not giving them the same attention. That's one more reason to try not to treat the child with epilepsy any differently from his brothers and sisters.

Brothers and sisters may show their feelings by picking on the child whom they resent, or they may try to win their parents' approval by copying them and pampering the child. Either reaction will be bad for the child with epilepsy, as well as for the other children.

When parents treat all their children the same way, they encourage a normal, healthy give-and-take between the brothers and sisters.

Some special treatment is inevitable. The child with epilepsy will probably visit the doctor more often, for example. So it's a good idea for parents to spend some time alone with the other children in the family. Let them talk about their feelings. They may feel guilt or shame about the epilepsy—or fear that they may get it. Family discussions about epilepsy allow all the children to bring their feelings into the open, where they can be dealt with realistically.

But My Other Relatives Say . . .

With other relatives—grandparents, uncles, aunts, cousins, etc.—the problem often is that they are too protective of the child with epilepsy. If this is happening in your family, have a quiet talk with your relatives. Explain to them that their behavior is not in the child's best interests.

It may be hard for them to change; but the effects will be minimal as long as you yourself treat the child as a normal, healthy, and responsible member of the family.

HOW WILL HE DO IN SCHOOL?

Teacher Pat Richards gave her Omaha sixth-graders an unusual learning experience recently. When one of her pupils had a mild seizure in school, Ms. Richards decided to teach her class the facts about epilepsy. With the help of

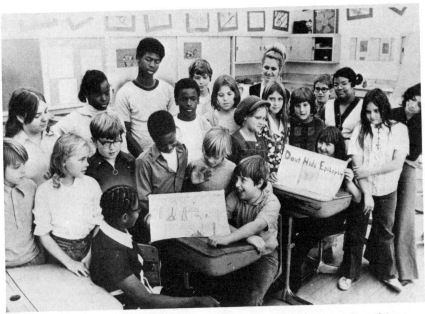

Pat Richards and class (*Omaha World-Herald* photograph by S. J. Melingagio).

the Nebraska Epilepsy League, she brought films and guest speakers to the class. The boys and girls even had a contest to see who could design the best poster about epilepsy.

Ms. Richards first learned about epilepsy when she was an education student at the University of Nebraska. It was a required part of her course—and it helped her become the kind of teacher all of us hope for.

Can My Child Go to a Regular School?

Most children with epilepsy go to regular public schools. They attend regular classes and take part in the classroom and extracurricular activities with the other children.

Few seizures are so severe that a child needs special education. But there are some children with more than one handicap—with multiple disabilities—whose needs a regular classroom situation cannot meet. Such children may be transferred to a special health class within the regular school—perhaps only for a short time, until the difficulties clear up. Or sometimes a child's parents may prefer to send him to a special school to better meet his needs.

Special Schools

For those few children whose needs cannot be adequately met by ordinary public, private, or parochial schools, there are schools equipped to deal with special problems—learning disabilities, emotional or behavioral problems, and so forth. The Epilepsy Foundation of America can supply you with information about such schools.

There is also the *Registry of Private Schools for Children with Special Education Needs,* compiled by the National Educational Consultant, Inc., and the *Directory of Residential Facilities for the Mentally Retarded* (this book includes schools for neurologically handicapped children who are not mentally retarded), compiled by the American Association of Mental Deficiency, the Special Education Information Center, and the Association for Children with Learning Disabilities. These two directories include admission criteria, programs, and fees for the schools they list.

Before deciding on any private school, investigate it carefully to see whether it meets the needs of your child. Visit the school and talk to the teachers. Speak to other parents about it, and check their experiences. Phone your local Epilepsy Foundation chapter, they may have some information about it.

Be sure that all your questions are answered and that you feel confident that this is the right school for your child.

Nursery Schools

Nursery schools are excellent ways of introducing a preschool child to a classroom situation. Don't overprotect your child with epilepsy by keeping him out. Meet the challenge of beating epilepsy from the first day it becomes known; this is the only way of conquering it.

Public day-care centers and nursery schools, as well as most private ones, accept children with epilepsy. So does Head Start, the Federal program for disadvantaged or handicapped preschoolers (ages three to five). By law, Head Start programs must have an enrollment of 10 percent handicapped children. To find out about eligibility, contact your local Head Start office or your local community action agency.

Camps

If seizures are under control, most camps, public or private, will accept children with epilepsy into their regular programs, especially if a doctor supports the application.

The child whose seizures are not controlled can also go to summer camp. There are special camps for handicapped children. The camp director, with the help of your physician, can evaluate your child's needs.

The Easter Seal Society, through its various regional affiliates, operates a number of camps throughout the country for children with all kinds of disabilities. Contact your local Easter Seal Society office for more information.

Many Epilepsy Foundation chapters also hold camps, or know of ones that will accept children with epilepsy. Also, the Camp Information Service, your local social service department, or your community health council should be able to provide you with others.

What Should I Tell the Teachers?

It's important to let the school or camp know that your child has epilepsy. In that way teachers will be prepared to handle any problems that may arise. There's a chance that your child, even if his seizures are well controlled, may have a seizure in class. If this happens, it helps for parents and teachers to have a prior understanding about what to do. A carefully made plan at the beginning of the school year is fairer to both the teacher and the child.

Be prepared to deal with some teachers' apprehension and lack of knowledge about epilepsy. Have an educational packet with you that is especially prepared for teachers by the Epilepsy Foundation. Take along a statement from your physician for the school nurse.

School personnel can be helpful to the child with epilepsy in many ways. One California mother writes:

> The soccer coach, the basketball coach . . . and the marvelous boys who run the "Y-camp" all faithfully do their parts in allowing [my child] to live a free and relaxed life.
> The basketball coach calls an "equipment time out" so that his best guard can take a pill!

Local chapters of the Epilepsy Foundation of America are doing their part to help teachers and other school staff accept and cope with the child with epilepsy. Their School Alert programs supply literature, films, posters, lesson plans, and other teaching aids about epilepsy to school personnel. It was through such a program that Ms. Richards got the materials she needed to teach her class about epilepsy. This sort of teaching is important because it takes the mystery and the stigma out of epilepsy.

Children who know the true facts about epilepsy will not consider the child who has it strange or different. And a child who is accepted is on the road to good adjustment.

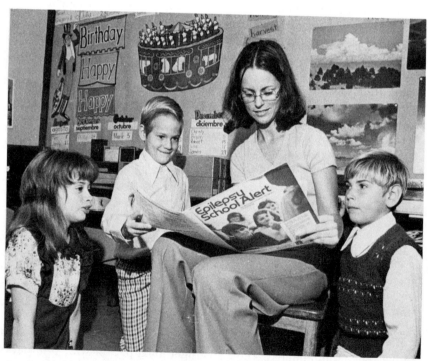

The EFA's School Alert programs provide materials for teaching children about epilepsy (*Tampa Tribune* photograph by Dan Fager).

Will My Child Have Trouble Learning?

Like any group of children, children with epilepsy have a wide range of learning ability. Many children with epilepsy are excellent students. Epilepsy does not cause learning disorders.

In some cases, though, learning handicaps may go along with epilepsy. For example, if the epilepsy is caused by a disorder in a particular part of the brain, the child's ability to process language or math information may be impaired. If the damaged cells are in the regions of the brain that control hearing, or memory, or integrating verbal instructions, or reading—or any of the individual brain processes that make learning possible—then a specific type of learning may be more difficult.

Not all learning difficulties are caused by damaged cells. Sometimes the problems can be caused by the very medicines that are used to control the disorder. Some anticonvulsants may have sedative side effects—they may slow a person down, and this sometimes has the effect of slowing down the learning processes as well. Other anticonvulsants may have the opposite effect—they sometimes make the person abnormally active (hyperactive), too much so to concentrate on learning.

On the other hand, uncontrolled epilepsy can also cause learning difficulties. The symptoms of petit mal epilepsy, for example, include frequent but very brief spells of unconsciousness. During these seizures, the child is unaware of what is going on around him, and afterwards he doesn't even realize that his consciousness was interrupted. He just goes on with whatever he was doing beforehand. This may cause trouble, because if the seizure has taken place during a lesson the child has no idea of what he was expected to learn. And a teacher who is unaware of his condition and what has happened may interpret his behavior as deliberate inattention. That's another reason for letting your child's teacher know about his condition.

Many schools have specially trained teachers to work with children with learning handicaps. These teachers can do a lot to help such children overcome their difficulties.

Will My Child Have Friends?

When children have been taught the facts about epilepsy, they are more likely to accept the child who has it. And when the child with epilepsy is kept in the mainstream of activities, he makes friends, as other children do. This is especially true when the child accepts himself and his condition, and when he is willing to deal with the challenge even when the going gets rough. Hope is the key.

Will Youth Groups Take My Child?

If a child's friends are joining the Boy Scouts or Girl Scouts or another youth group, he or she will want to join, too—and they should. This is an excellent way to keep in the mainstream of life and to learn the social skills and interpersonal relationships that are vital for good adjustment.

The national policy of the Girl Scouts, Boy Scouts, YMCA, YWCA, and church and synagogue groups is to encourage all children to join and to accept handicapped children into ordinary, nonhandicapped groups. However, on the local level, some groups may not always be aware of the national policy. If your child has trouble joining a local branch of a national organization, write to the national headquarters for assistance.

If your child has trouble joining a purely local group, contact your Epilepsy Foundation chapter for advice and help.

WHAT WILL THE TEEN YEARS BE LIKE?

The teen years are a time of changes. The body grows and develops. New sexual urges come into being. New schools are attended, new friendships are formed. And epilepsy must now be dealt with in a new context—taking into consideration the teenager's growing independence.

Growing Up

The changes that come during adolescence are hard for everybody to adjust to. There's a natural anxiety about separating oneself from the family. Many teenagers are tempted to hang on to their childhood a little bit longer, just for the sake of security. But this is false security; everybody has to grow up sometime. It may take the teenager with epilepsy a little longer to master this phase of development—he does have more to adjust to. So encourage him to take the first steps toward independence. It's a good idea to let him go away to school or camp if he wants to . . . to get an after-school job . . . to drive a car if he can get a license . . . to be as much like other teenagers as possible.

Epilepsy May Change, Too

Epilepsy sometimes changes during adolescence. Sometimes seizures stop altogether. Sometimes the type of seizure changes from petit mal to grand mal. And for many people, puberty is when seizures occur for the first time.

All these changes—like everything else about epilepsy—should be dealt with openly by both the parents and the teenager, so that they won't interfere—or will interfere only minimally—with the adolescent's normal development. Shame and secrecy just hide the problem and sometimes complicate it to a point where other problems may result; they don't make the disorder disappear.

Why Should I Be Different?

It's normal for teenagers to want to be just like their friends and to resent anything that sets them apart from the group. To some teenagers, this need is so urgent that they unwittingly deny, even to themselves, that they have epilepsy.

Denial is an unconscious attempt to solve a problem by denying that it exists. Of course, it doesn't really solve anything. Any problem you don't face up to will make adjustment—to school, to work, to interpersonal relationships—more difficult.

When you pretend you don't have epilepsy, you can also get into serious trouble medically. If you stop taking your medicine without your doctor's consent, you may have more frequent and severe seizures than ever before. You may even get into the dangerous state of status epilepticus.

If denial is a problem for you or your child, psychological advice may help. Adolescents with epilepsy and their parents can often benefit from some counseling. The school psychologist or your family doctor may be able to direct you to a counseling resource.

What About My Social Life?

The teen years are a time for dating and partying, and the teenager with epilepsy should join in the fun. But will people understand about your epilepsy?

Be prepared for the question to come up. Be able to talk about it. People don't know much about epilepsy—they may have all sorts of weird ideas on the subject. Hopefully, your friends will admire your frank, outspoken attitude, and you will serve as a model for them—but it may take a lot of persuasion, and you may need help in educating them.

It isn't easy. Some people are so set in their ways that you won't be able to change them—at least not immediately—no matter what you do. But try not to get too down about it. You may have to seek out those who can learn to understand, who can master the challenge, and who will value you as their friend.

Teen Groups

The Epilepsy Foundation of America sponsors groups where teenagers can get together with other teenagers with epilepsy to talk about their mutual problems. This is a good way to learn about epilepsy. It's also a good place to exchange experiences with others and see what solutions work in coping with epilepsy—in short, to work things out in a safe and accepting setting.

These groups are a good starting place, but they should not be your final destination. Don't try to use them to escape from people who don't have epilepsy, or from the natural stream of life.

How Can I Plan a Career?

Lots of teenagers find it hard to choose a career. For the teenager with epilepsy, the choice is twice as hard; he must consider not only his personal interests, abilities, needs, and values, but also any limitations that his disorder might impose. It would be foolish for anybody whose seizures are uncontrolled to plan a career which would put him or other people in danger; and it would be equally unwise to plan for a career—like the military—to which he would not be admitted because of his disorder.

However, it is not only the person with epilepsy who has this problem. Many people have some physical limitation on the work they can do. Nearsighted people don't become airline pilots—people who fear heights don't become steeplejacks.

So plan ahead for a career that's right for you. Ask around—but be sure that your advisers are knowledgeable about epilepsy. Vocational advisers at school can give you information about careers in general. Your doctor can give you data about your prognosis—his forecast of your health in future years—and this information can help you reach a decision. The Division of Vocational Rehabilitation also has prevocational counseling services.

Can I Go to College?

Of course you can go to college—if you are otherwise qualified to do so. Colleges and universities accept students with epilepsy.

Most colleges will require assurance from the student's doctor that he is receiving medical care. They will also want to know if any special arrangements are necessary for the student's safety. For example, can he work in a chemistry or physics lab? Can he use the gym? Can he live alone in the dormitory, or will he need a roommate?

Once these practical arrangements are settled, your success in college depends only on you.

FACTS AND FIGURES

How Many Children Have Epilepsy?

It is estimated that more than 2 million children in the United States have had a convulsive seizure. A significant percentage of these children later develop recurrent seizures and are considered to have epilepsy.

How Well Adjusted Are Children with Epilepsy?

In a 1972 survey, 41 percent of parents told the Epilepsy Foundation of America that their children with epilepsy were well adjusted. Another 23 percent noted occasional problems. Only 12 percent indicated extreme difficulty.

What Legislation Do Parents of Children with Epilepsy Want Most?

In the same survey, 59 percent of parents opted for medical research funding as the legislation that would help their children most.

5

Where to Find Help

WHO WILL HELP?

Sometimes it seems that nobody cares. But in fact there are many people who are trained to help the person with epilepsy—medically, psychosocially, and vocationally. All of the following professions may be involved in the care of people with epilepsy:

Family medicine specialists
General medical practitioners
Pediatricians
Neurologists
Neurosurgeons
Psychiatrists
Psychologists
Nurses
Social workers

Clinical laboratory technicians
EEG technologists
Hospital administrators
Vocational rehabilitation
  counselors
Employment specialists
Teachers and guidance
  counselors
Researchers

The Family Medicine Specialist or General Medical Practitioner

The family medicine specialist or general medical practitioner—the family doctor, in other words—often has a vital role to play in caring for the person with epilepsy. Often he is the first to diagnose the disorder. Usually the general practitioner is someone the family has consulted for a long time, and so he is familiar with the person's condition and will notice any changes that may signal possible neurologic problems.

Epilepsy isn't unusual. Most general practitioners have had some experience with it. Often they'll bring in a specialist for consultation and to confirm the diagnosis. Then, after a treatment regimen is arrived at and seizure control is established, the general practitioner will often continue follow-along management of the patient.

The Pediatrician

Pediatrics is the branch of medicine that is concerned with the health and development of the child. Because about two thirds of all epilepsy occurs before the age of 14, the pediatrician plays a very important role in epilepsy diagnosis and treatment. He is often the first doctor to be consulted when a first seizure occurs to someone in this age group.

Many pediatricians can handle the medical management of the child with epilepsy. In more complicated cases, they will often consult with a neurologist.

The Neurologist

A neurologist is a doctor who has had specialized training in the disorders of the brain and nervous system. Epilepsy is a disorder of the nervous system, so it falls within the neurologist's special field of competence. Neurologists are experienced in treating all types and variations of epilepsy, and they are able to make an accurate diagnosis quickly and provide adequate treatment at an early stage.

Sometimes a person consults a neurologist or an epileptologist (a doctor with a special interest in epilepsy) directly. More often, his family doctor, internist (a specialist in internal medicine), pediatrician, or another physician calls in the neurologist for consultation. The neurologist works closely with all these doctors, for a team of different specialists may be required to deal with all the aspects of epilepsy, social as well as medical. Unless the disorder is treated at the time of onset and is rapidly controlled without other factors entering in, treating seizures as a separate phenomenon neglects the disorder of epilepsy—the whole person must be treated if we are to achieve a full adjustment to epilepsy and a productive life.

If there is no neurologist in your community, your family doctor will know where you can obtain any clinical tests, examinations, or neurologic consultations that are necessary.

The Neurosurgeon

A neurosurgeon is a doctor who specializes in surgery on the brain and nervous system. In epilepsy, he might be called in to decide, in consultation with the rest of the medical team, whether brain surgery would be advisable.

There are a few centers that have a special interest in brain surgery as related to epilepsy. These include the University of Washington in Seattle and the Montreal Neurological Institute of McGill University.

The Psychiatrist

A psychiatrist is a doctor who specializes in treating mental and emotional disturbances. In many cases he is a member of the team of specialists who are helping the person with epilepsy.

The psychiatrist is involved in the overall adjustment of the person. He helps the patient deal with the emotional consequences of epilepsy and work these things through so that they don't become a barrier to normal living.

In fact, the whole team effort ideally should be directed to helping the person with epilepsy achieve the greatest degree of seizure control and as normal a lifestyle as possible.

The Psychologist

As more emphasis is given to problems in family and daily living and relations with other people, the clinical psychologist is becoming more and more involved with the problems of epilepsy.

Clinical psychologists diagnose, treat, and counsel people with emotional disorders. In epilepsy, this can mean helping the person deal with his feelings about seizures, and helping him overcome any other difficulties the disorder may cause in his life. The general public's lack of understanding of epilepsy and the economic and vocational problems faced by people with it can be real problems and can cause real distress. Psychologic counseling can help people deal realistically with the problems.

Besides clinical psychologists, there are other psychology specialists who can help people with epilepsy, for example, school psychologists and social psychologists.

School psychologists can help children make the most of their abilities. They can help identify and correct learning disabilities. They can interpret epilepsy to teachers and school administrators.

Social psychologists can study the relationships between people with epilepsy and other people in the community. Their findings may suggest ways to change public attitudes and eliminate stigma.

The Nurse

The nurse's role in the diagnosis, evaluation, and management of the patient with epilepsy is a supporting one. A hospital nurse may be the first person to see a seizure occur, and the nurse's observations can be important contributions to diagnosis. In the community, it is often the school nurse who first recognizes the symptoms of epilepsy in a child. The nurse is thus in an ideal position to work with the family, the doctor, and the school, for she can explain the problem to other students and to school personnel, prevent

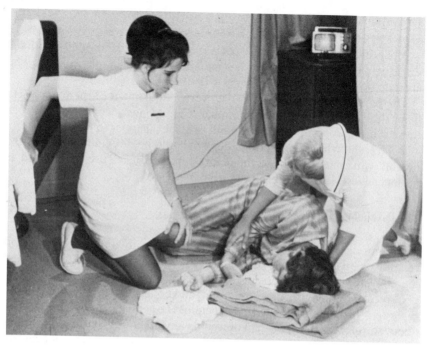

Nurses helping a person with epilepsy.

unwarranted program restrictions for the child, and gain understanding and acceptance for him.

Office nurses and public health nurses as well as school nurses are often in an excellent position to let the doctor know how well the person is reacting to his medicine. The nurse can help the family and the child with epilepsy by interpreting the sometimes confusing complexities that they are experiencing.

Patients and parents alike may sometimes appreciate talking to a nurse and feel less pressured about using the busy time of the doctor, although good doctors welcome parents' and childrens' questions.

The Social Worker

Social workers can help people whose epilepsy is causing problems. The social worker deals with the community as well as with individuals. From the person with epilepsy, his family, and his medical team, the social worker finds out just what that person needs and which of his needs are unmet. Then the social worker works with community groups—schools, employers, and so on—to try to get the needs satisfied.

A large part of the social work job is to help the community understand just what the individual's problems are and how they can be solved. By interpreting the needs of his clients with epilepsy, the social worker is helping to improve public understanding of this disorder.

Social workers are equipped to deal with emotional consequences as well as to offer concrete help.

The Clinical Laboratory Technician

Laboratory technicians include blood technicians, gas-liquid chromatography (GLC) technicians, and various other specialists. They are trained to do clinical tests in their specialty, such as blood tests, spinal tests, and x-rays. All these tests help the physician diagnose and treat the patient.

The EEG Technologist

EEG technologists are trained to record electroencephalograms—the brainwave recordings that are such valuable tools in diagnosing epilepsy.

The Hospital Administrator

Hospital administrators can help the person with epilepsy by helping to see that hospitals and clinics are effectively run so that the delivery of services by the hospital and professional staff is of top quality, and by being aware of the needs of people with epilepsy so that they can be included in hospital programs.

The Vocational Rehabilitation Counselor and the Employment Specialist

Vocational rehabilitation counselors and employment specialists are employed by government or private agencies. They are trained to assess the abilities and capabilities of a person and help match them with the jobs available in the labor market. These specialists can give a person realistic advice about his present or future career. They may help him to get further vocational training, or, through their contacts with employers in the community and their interpretation of epilepsy to these employers, they may be able to help the person with epilepsy get and keep a job.

The Teacher and the Guidance Counselor

The seeds of self-acceptance and community acceptance are sown in the classroom as well as at home. Teachers can help the child with seizures adjust to the problem. Equally important, they can help his classmates accept it. They serve as models for the children to follow.

Guidance counselors, too, can help with adjustment. And if these counselors are well informed about epilepsy, they can give helpful advice about choosing a career.

The Researcher

Researchers from all the relevant sciences and technical fields are constantly searching for new or improved ways to diagnose and treat epilepsy. They are also looking for the causes of epilepsy and for ways of preventing the disorder from occurring. When a course of treatment is discovered that will prevent seizures permanently—a cure—we will have the researchers to thank for it.

The Team

Government and private health authorities agree that the best way to treat people with epilepsy would be in multidisciplinary centers staffed by clinical teams of all the specialists we've listed above.

There are a few places like that in this country—at the University of Minnesota in Minneapolis, the Good Samaritan Hospital in Portland, Oregon, the University of Virginia in Charlottesville, the University of Washington in Seattle, and the Medical College of Georgia in Augusta. These facilities are called comprehensive epilepsy program centers and are funded by NINCDS which plans to establish more centers in the future.

There are also a number of seizure units at hospitals and medical centers throughout the country. These seizure units use a multidisciplinary team of neurologists, psychologists, psychiatrists, social workers, and counselors to help the person with epilepsy and his family. The Epilepsy Foundation of America publishes a directory of clinical facilities specializing in the treatment of epilepsy.

One of the goals of the epilepsy movement is to make the delivery of comprehensive epilepsy care a true team effort.

Volunteers

Paul E. Funk, former executive vice-president of the Epilepsy Foundation of America, has stated, "The problems of epilepsy, like most of the problems of our society, will be solved only by concerned citizens working together. Voluntarism is a primary American characteristic, and volunteers are still our one best hope for society."

Volunteers can help the person with epilepsy in just as many ways as their skills allow. Doctors, lawyers, salespeople, bankers, business men and women, students, retirees—all are volunteers, and all have some service to offer the person with epilepsy.

Most volunteers in the field of epilepsy work through the national voluntary organization, the Epilepsy Foundation of America, and its local and state chapters. It is the volunteers who make local chapter programs possible. As Paul Holland, attorney and former chairman of the board of the foundation, puts it, "EFA chapters are providing more services to more people with more skill than at any time, and several of them are approaching a professionalism that would do credit to any of our nation's major voluntaries."

There are also two international organizations concerned with epilepsy: the International Bureau for Epilepsy and the International League against Epilepsy.

The International Bureau for Epilepsy (IBE) is primarily concerned with the social and economic problems of people who have epilepsy. The Epilepsy Foundation of America belongs to the IBE. So do seventeen other national lay organizations in foreign countries, and fifteen epilepsy institutions.

Waging the battle on the professional level are organizations of physicians and scientists concerned with the medical and psychosocial aspects of epilepsy. They are affiliated with the International League against Epilepsy (ILE). The American Epilepsy Society, an organization of physicians and neuroscientists—mostly neurologists—and other professionals concerned with finding and applying new knowledge about epilepsy, is a member of the ILE.

Government

"I believe that all Americans have the right to expect their government to take all reasonable and prudent steps to deliver or set them free from the 'evil' of epilepsy," Ellen R. Grass, senior vice-president of the Epilepsy Foundation of America, stated in testimony before the House Subcommittee on Health in 1974. And government does play a part in helping people with epilepsy. We have already discussed some of the agencies that help. Another law that is helpful is the Developmental Disabilities Services and Facilities Construction Act.

This act is used to provide Federal funds for state programs in epilepsy, as well as other developmental disabilities. The act defines a developmental disability as one that (1) originates before a person reaches the age of eighteen; (2) has continued or can be expected to continue indefinitely; and (3) constitutes a substantial handicap. The act has been used to fund a wide range of services—educational, vocational, and rehabilitational.

To make government services even more efficient, leaders in the epilepsy movement have been calling for a national plan for the control of epilepsy. Paul E. Funk says, "The resources of the entire nation must be mobilized, and a national plan to guide local programs is an urgent need."

Former Representative Peter N. Kyros of Maine, in calling for such a national plan, said that it would be "a major achievement—a milestone in the true sense of the word—for the epilepsy movement." He adds, "This is a problem of such size and scope, affecting so many aspects of human relationships, that there is more than enough room for all of us to pitch in and help."

In 1975, Congress recognized the need for national action when it established a national commission to study epilepsy and make recommendations for its control. This Commission for the Control of Epilepsy and Its Consequences includes many distinguished epileptologists; its Chairman, Dr. David D. Daly, is well aware of the problems of epilepsy. The Commission's report to Congress has now been completed. Thus, we have moved one step closer toward a national plan.

The Person with Epilepsy

Through collective action, people with epilepsy and their families can be their own best helpers. By getting involved with other concerned people in the epilepsy movement—by spreading the word in the community—by volunteering their services in hospitals, rehabilitation centers, and epilepsy associations—by speaking up for themselves—they can help to overcome their own problems. And this is the way in which the problems of epilepsy will finally be solved.

Epilepsy is a community problem as well as an individual and a family problem, and its solution depends on action on all three levels.

WHERE CAN I TURN?

Actually, in most communities there are a lot of services available from public and private agencies for people with epilepsy. But the red tape involved in finding the proper resource can be very hard to unwind. It would help if there were information and referral services to tell people where in their community to go for assistance with a particular problem. In communities where there is a chapter of the Epilepsy Foundation of America, that office would be the first place to check for referral information. If there is no chapter in your community, finding help requires a bit more effort.

Where to Go for What

The table on pages 93 and 94 lists services that people with epilepsy may need, along with the principal public and private agencies that supply such services in most communities.

To find a specific public or private agency, contact your local health and welfare council. Always check first to see if there is an Epilepsy Foundation of America chapter in your community, for they will be able to give you helpful advice.

Community Services for People with Epilepsy

Service Needed	Where to Find it
Clinics	Local department of public health Medical centers Medical schools State department of mental hygiene State department of public health State medical society Teaching hospitals
Dental	Crippled children's services Dental school Local department of public health Medical centers State dental society State department of public health Teaching hospitals
Education	Local department of education State crippled children's services State department of education Universities or colleges of education
Employment and Vocational	State department of vocational rehabilitation State employment service United States Employment Service
Extended care	Local council of social agencies Local department of public health State department of public health
Family	Local department of public welfare, family services division
Financial	Crippled children's service Family Association of America Local department of public welfare Salvation Army Social Security office State department of vocational rehabilitation
Health	*See* Clinics
Hospitals	Local department of public health Local hospital association Veterans' Administration
Housing	Local department of public welfare Salvation Army
Legal	American Civil Liberties Union Legal defender (in Massachusetts) Local Legal Aid office Public defender service University school of law

Community Services for People with Epilepsy—*Continued*

Service Needed	*Where to Find It*
Medicines	Crippled children's service Medicaid Medicare
Nursing	Local department of public health State department of public health Visiting Nurses Association
Psychologic, psychiatric	American Psychological Association Community mental health clinics Local mental health service Local psychology and/or psychiatry association State department of mental hygiene State psychology and/psychiatry association
Recreation	Local department of recreation State department of recreation YMCA-YWCA YMHA-YWHA
Residential	Department of public welfare Local council of social agencies Private facilities
Sheltered and transitional workshops	State department of vocational rehabilitation
Transportation	Local department of public welfare Red Cross transportation program State crippled children's service
Volunteers	Epilepsy Foundation of America chapter Local department of public welfare Red Cross volunteer programs

How Can I Find a Neurologist?

Your family doctor can direct you to an epileptologist when necessary. If you do not have a family doctor, ask your local Epilepsy Foundation chapter for a list of specialists in your community who have an interest in epilepsy.

If you live in a rural area, ask the public health nurse about how to get medical services in your vicinity. The public health nurse is usually listed in the telephone directory under city or county government.

Should I Go to a Clinic?

In some communities, there are special seizure clinics for the diagnosis and treatment of epilepsy. Such clinics are usually part of a hospital or medical center and offer the services of a large staff of competent doctors and other personnel. Their treatment is on an outpatient basis—that is, the person does not have to be admitted to the hospital. Many clinics base their fees on the patient's income.

Your local health department can help you find a clinic. If you are a veteran and you developed epilepsy in the service, consult your local Veterans' Administration hospital. Also, a list of clinics that serve people with epilepsy is available from the Epilepsy Foundation of America.

Will I Have to Go to the Hospital?

Epilepsy is usually diagnosed and treated on an outpatient basis. But there are times when a person might need in-hospital care. There are some special diagnostic procedures and treatments that just can't be done at home, at a clinic, or in a doctor's office. A person is hospitalized when:

1. He has a prolonged grand mal seizure, or a grand mal seizure followed immediately by another without recovering consciousness in-between. This is status epilepticus—a major medical emergency that requires special therapy and general intensive care in a hospital to end the attack.
2. His seizures are not controlled and do not seem to respond to anticonvulsant medicines. If the person is hospitalized, his medication can be carefully observed and supervised to see if an effective combination and dosage can be reached.
3. There are neurologic symptoms that can't be accounted for. In a hospital, extensive studies not otherwise possible can be done in order to find out what's causing the problem.
4. It's necessary, for diagnosis and treatment, for medical people to observe the seizures. Close observation and electronic monitoring procedures can produce information that is valuable for diagnosis and treatment.

Do Mental Hospitals Treat Epilepsy?

Epilepsy is a neurologic disorder, not an emotional illness. Therefore, it is treated in regular hospitals, not in "mental" hospitals.

However, although epilepsy does not cause mental illness, there are some people who suffer from mental illness in addition to epilepsy. In such cases, a person might have to spend some time in a mental hospital for treatment of the mental illness. The patient's doctor will recommend a suitable mental hospital.

Are People with Epilepsy Institutionalized?

A few generations ago it was thought that residential institutions were the logical places to send people with severe chronic conditions that could not be treated or cured. Now there are still some institutions for such people, but it is generally recognized that it is better for most people to live in regular surroundings within the community. Even people who have severe and recurrent seizures are better off at home or in special day-care or residential-care facilities than in an institution.

If the person does not have a home to go to, and if he is unable to live alone, there are still alternatives to institutionalization in some communities.

New York City has pioneered foster homes for adults. The person who needs a home is matched with a person who wants to provide one. The program includes a staff of counselors for both parties. Other communities have adopted this type of program, too—Toledo, Ohio, for example.

In Virginia, a new program called Service Integration for Deinstitutionalization (SID) is setting up procedures to deinstitutionalize people by integrating them into the community.

In addition, the US Department of Health, Education, and Welfare (HEW) has funded projects called Community Alternatives to Institutionalization and Institutional Reform (CAIR) to help states devise better methods for helping disabled people.

Do Nursing Homes Accept People with Epilepsy?

Epilepsy can add to the other problems of old age. For one thing, the bones of elderly people are fragile, and to prevent broken legs or arms the elderly person with epilepsy has to be protected from getting hurt in a seizure.

A suitable nursing home for the older person with epilepsy is one that has an enlightened staff and administrators who understand epilepsy and its nursing needs. Whether a nursing home will accept a particular individual with epilepsy depends on the home's understanding of epilepsy and on the individual's degree of seizure control and freedom from other complicating problems.

Your doctor or the social service department at the hospital should be able to help you find a suitable nursing home.

Can I Get a Discount on Medicine?

It is important to take anticonvulsant medicine in the precise doses that your doctor prescribes. There are several ways of obtaining reliable medicines at a lower cost:

1. By buying in bulk. If your prescription doesn't change, you can usually save money by buying a lot of it at once. In some states, however, there may be restrictions on the amount you can buy at one time.
2. By asking for a medicine by its generic name, not its brand name. Medicines are generally cheaper if you buy them by their generic name instead of by the name given to them by one or other of the companies that manufacture them. The generic names of the anticonvulsants are shown in the table on page 27.

   But be careful: the Food and Drug Administration has found that not all brands of anticonvulsants have the same effect. Ask your doctor's opinion; you can't buy a drug under its generic name unless your doctor writes it that way in the prescription.
3. By comparison shopping. Prices of prescription drugs often vary from one drugstore to the next. Shop around; prices generally aren't advertised, but the druggist should tell them to you if you phone or visit the store.
4. Through state programs. Some states have tax-supported programs whereby medicines can be purchased more cheaply. Ask your department of health whether your state has such a program.
5. Through Medicare or Medicaid. Contact your local Social Security office to find out if you are eligible for these programs.
6. Through the Epilepsy Foundation of America. The EFA has established a Prescription Drug Program through which members may purchase prescription medicine at a discount. Ask your local chapter or write EFA headquarters for details of the plan.

Can I Get Medicine through the Mail?

There are places that fill prescriptions by mail. Sometimes you can get medicine at a discount this way—the EFA's Prescription Drug Program is a mail-order program. You may find shopping by mail more convenient, even without a discount, particularly if you live in a rural area.

Many reliable, well-known clinics and pharmacies issue medicine through the mail. On the other hand, there are some mail-order firms that are not reliable. Their medicines are not what your doctor prescribed. They may contain only a small amount of anticonvulsants, and so they are of limited value.

Check out any mail-order drug company very carefully before ordering from it. Even if the firm is reliable, remember that you must plan ahead when you order. Leave enough time so that you do not run out of the drug if the mail is delayed; a sudden withdrawal from your medicine may bring on seizures. And be prepared to throw out unused medicines if your prescription changes.

Can I Get Financial Help?

There are several agencies that give financial help to some people with epilepsy. Your local and state departments of public welfare will have detailed information on local, state, and Federal assistance in your community. Because services and eligibility requirements vary from area to area, it is a good idea to consult both these departments.

If you need short-term help, try the Family Association of America. In some areas of the country, this agency's offices maintain funds to help out in emergency situations.

For financial aid for work training, try the Division of Vocational Rehabilitation. If, in their opinion, further education is consistent with your abilities and will help you achieve your job goals, they may help.

For information about Social Security benefits, see pages 67 and 68.

HOW CAN I HELP?

The person who can do the most for the person with epilepsy is . . . himself. If you have epilepsy, you can help yourself by:

Keeping healthy.
Taking an active part in life.
Joining your efforts with those of others who want to combat epilepsy.

Keeping Healthy

You owe it to yourself to keep as healthy as possible. This includes following your doctor's advice, having regular checkups, and not neglecting to take your medicine.

This is your responsibility to yourself, your family, and your community.

Taking an Active Part in Life

It is also your responsibility to take an active part in life. Every human being has problems. Withdrawal is not the answer.

Nobody is going to drag you out of the closet; come out yourself, and join the action.

Joining with Others

By joining the fight against epilepsy, you can take an active part in solving your own problems.

"The time has come for you to step forward," says Paul E. Funk, former executive vice-president of EFA. Volunteers are needed in every phase of the struggle against epilepsy. They are needed to raise funds, to work with other people who have epilepsy, to do clerical work; to help in chapter administration, to see that Federal and state budgets adequately fund epilepsy programs, and to give advice in their own areas of expertise. Everybody has some contribution to make.

One phase of volunteer work that needs greater emphasis and deserves wider recognition and appreciation is the raising of funds. Without money there can be no research, no social programs, no public information effort. For this reason, the comments of Thomas A. O'Neil, J.D., C.P.A., and treasurer of the Epilepsy Foundation of America, are particularly worth noting: "An encouraging development is the increase in revenue generated by our chapter network. If this growth continues, chapters will eventually be able to assume a more equitable share of funding responsibility, which, on an overall basis, has until now been borne mostly by the national office."

To volunteer, contact your local chapter or your regional office of the Epilepsy Foundation of America; they need you.

The Foundation

Another way to help is to become a member of the Epilepsy Foundation of America. James M. Watson, M.D., of the foundation's board of directors, has this to say about the membership program:

It offers concerned laymen and professionals an opportunity to join the epilepsy movement while providing more meaningful services to members who have epilepsy themselves or in their families. The program will offer new members both national and local services, including information on low-cost drug and insurance programs, basic materials on epilepsy, and the opportunity to contribute to—and benefit from—other local chapter activities.

So contact your local or state EFA office. Join your voice and influence to those of the thousands of other people in our country who have banded together to fight epilepsy.

FACTS AND FIGURES

How Many People Are Concerned with Epilepsy?

About 5 million. This includes people with epilepsy and their families, friends, coworkers, employers, employees, and neighbors; service workers, such as policemen; volunteers; and the professionals involved in epilepsy care.

How Many Volunteers Are There in the Epilepsy Movement?

About 30,000.

How Many More Volunteers Are Needed?

As many as possible.

Epilepsy Terms

Here are some brief definitions of some of the medical terms sometimes associated with epilepsy. For a more detailed list, see Gastaut, H.: *Dictionary of Epilepsy, Part I: Definitions.* World Health Organization, Geneva, 1973.

Abdominal Seizure. An epileptic seizure characterized by sensations in the abdomen.

Absence. A brief lowering or loss of consciousness.

Absence Status. A form of status epilepticus *(q.v.)* consisting of a prolonged or repeated absence.

Activation. A deliberate bringing on of a seizure for the purpose of studying it.

Acupuncture. A treatment involving puncturing the body.

Advocacy. The public promotion of a cause.

Affective. Having to do with mood or emotion.

Affective Seizure. (1) A seizure beginning with a feeling or emotion. (2) A seizure thought to be brought on by an emotion.

Air Study. Pneumoencephalogram.

Akinetic Seizure. A seizure characterized by falling and a loss of the ability to move.

Anemia. A blood deficiency condition.

Angiography. X-ray of blood vessels.

Anticonvulsant. A drug that prevents epileptic seizures.

Antiepileptic. Anticonvulsant.

Aphasic Seizure. A partial seizure characterized by temporary speech impairment.

Arteriography. X-ray of an artery or of the arterial system.

Asymptomatic Epilepsy. Epilepsy that cannot be linked to a definite cause.

Atonic. Characterized by a fall to the ground.

Attack. A sudden sickness. Also used to mean a seizure.

Auditory Seizure. A partial seizure in which the person hears sounds that are not present.

Aura. The first manifestation of a seizure. Sometimes used to mean a warning.

Automatic Seizure. A seizure characterized by involuntary movements.

Automatism. An involuntary activity.

Autonomic Effects. Internal changes in the body.

Autonomic System. A part of the nervous system controlling the so-called involuntary workings of the body.

Axon. The transmitting portion of the nerve cell.

Behavior Modification. A psychologic method that tries to change behavior by using immediate rewards and punishments.

Bilateral Massive Myoclonus. A brief, involuntary contraction affecting adjoining sets of muscles and thus causing turbulent movement.

Biofeedback. A technique of letting you see or hear your body processes so you can learn to change them.

Blood Level Testing. A laboratory method for measuring the amount of drug in the blood.

Brain. The mass of nerve tissue encased in the skull.

Brain Scan. A type of brain x-ray.

Brain Wave. The electrical activity of the brain.

Cataleptic Attack. A sudden loss of muscle tone; not used in relation to epilepsy.

Center of Excellence. An epilepsy treatment center staffed by clinical teams of specialists.

Central Nervous System. The brain and spinal cord.

Centrencephalic Epilepsy. Epilepsy in which the center of the brain is involved.

Cerebellum. A part of the brain responsible for the coordination of movements.

Cerebral Cortex. The outer layer of the brain.

Clinical Findings. The results of a physical examination and laboratory tests.

Clonic. Jerking.

Clonic Seizure. A seizure occurring in early infancy characterized by loss of consciousness, internal bodily symptoms, and jerking movements.

Clonus. In epilepsy, the jerking phase of a convulsive seizure.

Cognitive. Having to do with thoughts or ideas.

Coma. A state of deep unconsciousness.

Computerized Axial Tomographic Scan (CAT Scan). A computerized x-ray.

Conditioned Seizure. A seizure thought to be brought on by some factor the person has learned to associate with seizure symptoms.

Confusion. In epilepsy, a state of bewilderment that sometimes occurs during or immediately after a seizure.

Congenital. Existing at or before birth.

Convulsant. A drug that produces convulsions.

Convulsion. Any involuntary contraction of the muscles.

Convulsive. Characterized by or related to convulsions.

Convulsive Predisposition. A susceptibility to seizures.

Convulsive Threshold. The point at which a seizure can be produced.

Cortical Epilepsy. Epilepsy in which the nerve discharge causing the seizures is located in the cerebral cortex of the brain.

Craniotomy. An operation in which an opening is made in the skull.

Dendrite. The receiving portion of a nerve cell.

Denial. An unconscious attempt to solve a problem by denying that it exists.

Diagnosis. The identification of a disease or disorder.

Drop Attack. A seizure in which control of some muscles is temporarily lost.

Electroencephalograph. A machine that graphically records brain waves.

Epileptiform Seizure. A seizure that resembles epilepsy but whose cause is undetermined.

Epilepsy. A chronic brain disorder characterized by recurrent seizures.

Epileptic. Referring to epilepsy.

Epileptic Cry. A sound made during a seizure. It is caused by the passage of air through the respiratory tract.

Epileptic Discharge. A discharge of electricity in the brain caused by a large number of nerve cells being activated at the same time.

Epileptic Equivalent. An old term for seizures other than grand mal.

Epileptic Focus. (1) All the nerve cells involved in an epileptic discharge. (2) The nerve cells where the discharge originated.

Epileptic Personality. A term reflecting the mistaken belief that there are certain personality characteristics that accompany epilepsy.

Epileptic Predisposition. A susceptibility to epilepsy.

Epileptic Seizure Discharge. The brain wave pattern pictured on the electroencephalogram during seizures.

Epileptic Threshold. A measure of predisposition of a person with epilepsy for developing a seizure.

Epileptiform; Epileptoid. Similar to epilepsy.

Epileptogenic. Likely to cause epilepsy or an epileptic seizure.

Epileptogenic Focus. A brain injury at the site of which nerve cells discharge to cause a seizure.

Epileptologist. A physician specializing in epilepsy.

Epileptology. A branch of medicine concerned with epilepsy.

Essential Epilepsy. *See* Asymptomatic Epilepsy.

Evoked Seizure. A seizure regularly brought on by some definite factor.

Falling Sickness. Old term for epilepsy, especially for grand mal.

Familial Epilepsy. Epilepsy in several members of the same family.

Family Medicine Practitioner. A family doctor.

Febrile Convulsions. Convulsions occurring during fever.

Febrile Convulsions, Simple. Febrile convulsions that do not have aftereffects.

Febrile Epilepsy. Epilepsy triggered by episodes of fever.

Febrile Seizure. A seizure brought on by fever.

Fit. A seizure.

Focal Epilepsy. Partial epilepsy.

Frontal Epilepsy. Epilepsy in which the nerve discharge causing the seizures is located in the premotor frontal cortex of the brain.

Furor. A rare state of rage occurring after a seizure.

Gastrointestinal Reflex Seizure. *See* Gastrointestinal Seizure.

Gastrointestinal Seizure. An autonomic *(q.v.)* seizure with symptoms related to the digestive tract. *See also* Abdominal Seizure.

Generalized Seizure. A seizure with loss of consciousness and autonomic *(q.v.)* symptoms affecting both sides of the body at the same time.

General Medical Practitioner. A family doctor.

Generic Name. Nonproprietary name.

Genetic Epilepsy. Hereditary epilepsy.

Genuine Epilepsy. *See* Essential Epilepsy.

Grand Mal. (1) A tonic-clonic seizure. (2) Any type of epilepsy with major seizures.

Gray Matter. The nerve tissue of the brain.

Gustatory Seizure. A partial seizure characterized by sensations of tastes that are not actually present.

Hallucination. Something that is perceived through the senses but that isn't really there.

Hepatitis. A liver disorder.

Hyperactivity. Excessive activity.

Hyperexcitable. Easily aroused.

Hypertrophy. Extra growth.

Hyperventilation. A method of inducing a seizure by having the person breathe very rapidly.

Ictal. Relating to or happening during a seizure.

Idiopathic Epilepsy. Asymptomatic epilepsy.

Illusion. In epilepsy, an alteration of perception occurring in some partial seizures.

Infantile Convulsions. Convulsions in very young children.

Interictal. Interseizure.

Internist. A physician specializing in internal medicine.

Interseizure. Occurring between two seizures.

Intestinal Seizure. Abdominal seizure.

Intravenous. Injections made directly into the vein.

Ion. An electrically charged atom or group of atoms.

Jacksonian. An epileptic symptom that spreads along one side of the body.

Jacksonian Convulsions. Convulsions that start in one part of the body and spread to other parts.

Jacksonian March. The spread of a seizure from one muscle area to the next or from one skin area to the next.

Jaundice. A yellowing of the skin and tissues.

Ketogenic Diet. A high fat, low carbohydrate diet.

Lesion. A change in the body caused by injury or disease.

Major Seizure. A tonic-clonic seizure.

MCT Ketogenic Diet. Oil-based version of the ketogenic diet *(q.v.)*.

Menstrual Seizure. A seizure occurring during menstruation, or immediately before or after.

Migraine. A severe, recurrent headache, usually on one side of the head. Not a symptom of epilepsy.

Minor Seizure. A lesser seizure in people who also get grand mal seizures.

Motor. Having to do with motion.

Multiple Disabilities. More than one handicap.

Myoclonic Jerk. Bilateral massive myoclonus.

Myoclonic Seizure. (1) A very brief epileptic seizure characterized by involuntary muscle contractions on both sides of the body. (2) A series of involuntary muscle contractions recurring at short intervals over a period of a few seconds or minutes.

Myoclonus. A brief, involuntary muscle contraction.

Narcolepsy. A recurrent, uncontrollable urge to sleep. Not related to epilepsy.

Natal. At birth.

Neurochemistry. The study of chemical processes in the nervous system.

Neurologist. A physician specializing is disorders of the brain and nervous system.

Neurology. The study of the brain and nervous system.

Neuron. A nerve cell.

Neuronal Discharge. The electric potential that results from the activation of one or more neurons.

Neuropharmacology. The study of the effects of drugs on the nervous system.

Neurosurgeon. A brain surgeon.

Neurosurgery. Brain surgery.

Nocturnal Epilepsy. Epilepsy in which the seizures occur mainly at night, during sleep.

Olfactory Seizure. A seizure in which the person smells odors that are not actually present.

Parietal Epilepsy. Epilepsy in which the discharge causing the seizures is located in the parietal cortex of the brain.

Paroxysm. Convulsion.

Paroxysmal Convulsive Disorder. Epilepsy.

Partial Seizure. A seizure with symptoms that are not as extensive as those of a generalized seizure.

Pediatrician. A physician specializing in the care of children.

Petit Mal Seizure. (1) A seizure characterized by absence *(q.v.)* or myoclonus *(q.v.)*. (2) Any minor epileptic seizure.

Photic Stimulation. A method of inducing a seizure by having the person look at a flickering light.

Pneumoencephalography. A procedure whereby air is injected into the spinal cord. The air passes to the brain, and an x-ray is taken to show the air spaces.

Postictal. Postseizure.

Postseizure. After a seizure.

Post-Traumatic Epilepsy. Epilepsy due to a head injury.

Preictal. Preseizure.

Prenatal. Before birth.

Preseizure. Before a seizure.

Preseizure Epileptic Manifestations. Symptoms occurring before a seizure. (*Not* the aura, which is actually the beginning of a seizure.)

Prodrome. In epilepsy, symptoms occurring some time (from several hours to several days) before a seizure. Can serve as a warning.

Prognosis. A forecast of future health.

Psychiatrist. A physician specializing in the treatment of mental and emotional disorders.

Psychologist. A specialist in the study of mental processes and behavior.

Psychomotor Epilepsy. Temporal lobe epilepsy.

Recurrent Seizures. Seizures that occur again and again at intervals.

Rh Factor. A substance present in most people's red blood cells.

Sacred Disease. Old name for epilepsy.

Saint John's Disease. Old name for grand mal.

Saint Valentine's Disease. Old name for grand mal.

Seizure Threshold. A person's susceptibility toward the development of seizures.

Senses. Sight, hearing, smell, taste, and touch.

Sensory. Relating to the senses.

Skullplate. X-ray of the skull and brain.

Spasm. An involuntary muscle contraction.

Spike-And-Wave. A brain wave pattern characteristic of petit mal seizures.

Spinal Cord. The part of the nervous system that is encased in the backbone.

Status Epilepticus. A serious condition characterized by extremely prolonged or continuous seizures.

Stimulus. Anything that activates the brain or a sense organ.

Symptomatic Epilepsy. Epilepsy whose immediate cause can be proved.

Synchronous. In electroencephalography, a term meaning that all the electrical activity of the brain is locked into a single pattern.

Television Epilepsy. Epilepsy in which seizures are brought on by closely watching television in partial darkness. (*Not* a seizure that accidentally happens to occur while the person is watching TV.)

Temporal Lobe Epilepsy. Epilepsy in which the nerve discharge causing the seizures is located in the temporal lobe of the brain.

Tonic. Rigid.

Tonic-Clonic. The succession of rigid and jerking phases in a convulsive seizure.

Toxic. Harmful or poisonous.

Tumor. An abnormal growth.

Ventriculogram. X-ray of the brain cavities.

Bibliography

There have been scores of books published about epilepsy. There are also articles on epilepsy published in professional journals, general interest articles in magazines, and pamphlets and brochures on epilepsy published by the Epilepsy Foundation of America. The following is a list of books that are particularly helpful in explaining various facets of epilepsy. Many of these books are available in bookstores and in public libraries. If your library does not have them, you might be able to persuade your librarian to purchase at least one or two of them; or the librarian might arrange to borrow some books through an interlibrary loan from a Federal agency, such as the National Library of Medicine or the library of the Department of Health, Education, and Welfare. Other resources for borrowing books are medical school libraries, the libraries of large hospitals, or your local chapter of the Epilepsy Foundation of America.

General Books

Boshes, L. D. and Gibbs, F. A.: *Epilepsy Handbook,* ed. 2. Charles C Thomas, Springfield, Ill., 1972.
Lennox, W. G. and Lennox, M. A.: *Epilepsy and Related Disorders, 2 vols.* Little, Brown and Company, Boston, 1960.
Scott, D.: *About Epilepsy.* Gerald Duckworth, London, 1973.

Dictionaries

Gastaut, H.: *Dictionary of Epilepsy.* World Health Organization, Geneva, 1973.

The Child

Baird, H.: *The Child with Convulsions: A Guide for Parents, Teachers, Counselors, and Medical Personnel.* Grune & Stratton, New York, 1972.

Heisler, V.: *A Handicapped Child in the Family: A Guide for Parents.* Grune & Stratton, New York, 1972.

Jacksonville Epilteens: *Seizureology.* Tallahassee Developmental Disabilities Council, 1974. Distributed by Coordinator, Learning Resource Center, Division of Retardation, 1131 Winewood Blvd., Building 5, Tallahassee, Florida 32301.

Lagos, J. C.: *Seizures, Epilepsy, and Your Child.* Harper & Row, New York, 1974.

Livingston, S.: *Comprehensive Management of Epilepsy in Infancy, Childhood and Adolescence.* Charles C Thomas, Springfield, Ill., 1972.

Rehabilitation

Wright, G.: *Epilepsy Rehabilitation.* Little, Brown and Company, Boston, 1974.

History

Hippocrates: *Medical Works.* Trans. by Jones, W. H. S. Loeb Classical Library, Harvard University Press, Cambridge, Mass.

Temkin, O.: *The Falling Sickness: A History of Epilepsy from the Greeks to the Beginnings of Modern Neurology.* Johns Hopkins University Press, Baltimore, 1971.

Epilepsy Foundation of America Publications

The Epilepsy Foundation of America is constantly publishing new literature about epilepsy. A complete list of these publications may be obtained from the Epilepsy Foundation of America at 1828 L Street NW, Washington, D.C. 20036.

Index

113

Treatment of epilepsy—*Continued*
  anticonvulsant drugs and, 25–26
    actions of, 26–27
    addiction and, 31
    alcohol and, 31
    doctor-patient teamwork and, 32
    monitoring blood levels of, 27–28
    in animals, 32
    long-term effects of, 32
    other medicines in combination with, 29
    side effects of, 28–29
    when no longer needed, 32
  behavior modification and, 36
  biofeedback and, 35–36
  ketogenic diets and, 34
  surgery and, 33–34

Tumors, of brain, as cause of epilepsy, 17

UNCLASSIFIED seizures, 8
Unilateral seizures, 8, 10–11

VOCATIONAL counseling, 82, 89
Volunteers, 90–91

WILKS, Samuel, 26
Work. *See* Employment.
Workers' Compensation, 54

YOUTH groups, children with epilepsy and, 79–81
YMCA, children with epilepsy and, 80
YWCA, children with epilepsy and, 80